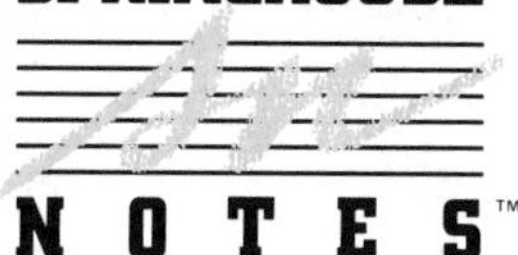

SPRINGHOUSE NOTES™

COMMUNITY HEALTH NURSING

Joan R. Howard, RN, EdD
Dr. Howard, the author of this book, is an Associate Professor of Nursing at Kean College, Union, N.J. She earned her BSN from the University of Michigan, Ann Arbor, her MSN from the University of Pennsylvania, Philadelphia, and her EdD from West Virginia University. Dr. Howard is a member of the American Nurses' Association, the New Jersey State Nurses' Association, the American Public Health Association, the New Jersey Public Health Association, the New Jersey Society of Public Health Educators, American Diabetes Association, and Sigma Theta Tau.

Kenny Mallow Williamson, RN, MSN
Ms. Williamson, the reviewer of this book, is an Instructor in the Community Health Nursing Graduate Program at the University of Alabama, Birmingham. She earned her BSN from Samford University, Birmingham, and her MSN from the University of Alabama, Birmingham. Ms. Williamson is a member of Sigma Theta Tau, the American Nurses' Association, the National League for Nursing, and the Association for Practitioners in Infection Control.

Springhouse Corporation
Springhouse, Pennsylvania

Staff

Executive Director, Editorial
Stanley Loeb

Executive Director, Creative Services
Jean Robinson

Director of Trade and Textbooks
Minnie B. Rose, RN, BSN, MEd

Art Director
John Hubbard

Consultant
Maryann Foley, RN, BSN

Acquisitions Editor
Donna L. Hilton, RN, BSN, CEN

Editors
Kevin Law (manager), Judd Howard

Copy Editors
David Prout (manager), Margaret MacKay Eckman, Elizabeth Kiselev

Designers
Stephanie Peters (associate art director), Julie Carleton Barlow

Art Production
Robert Perry (manager), Anna Brindisi, Donald Knauss, Catherine Mace, Robert Wieder

Typography
David Kosten (manager), Diane Paluba (assistant manager), Joyce Rossi Biletz, Brenda C. Mayer, Robin Rantz, Brent Rinedoller, Valerie L. Rosenberger

Manufacturing
Deborah Meiris (manager), T.A. Landis, Jennifer Suter

Production Coordination
Aline S. Miller (manager), Maura C. Murphy

The clinical procedures described and recommended in this publication are based on research and consultation with nursing, medical, and legal authorities. To the best of our knowledge, these procedures reflect currently accepted practice; nevertheless, they can't be considered universal recommendations. For individual application, all recommendations must be considered in light of the patient's clinical condition and, before administration of new or infrequently used drugs, in light of latest package-insert information. The authors and the publisher disclaim responsibility for any adverse effects resulting directly or indirectly from the suggested procedures, from any undetected errors, or from the reader's misunderstanding of the text.

Printed in the United States of America.

SN9-010789

Library of Congress Cataloging-in-Publication Data
Howard, Joan R.
Community health nursing.
(Springhouse notes)
Bibliography: p. Includes index.
1. Community health nursing—Outlines, syllabi, etc. I. Williamson, Kenny Mallow. II. Title. III. Series. [DNLM: 1. Community Health Nursing—outlines.
WY 18 H849c]
RT98.H69 1990 610.73′43 89-6031
ISBN 0-87434-204-X

Beverly's Book!

Contents

How to Use Springhouse Notes

Today, more than ever, nursing students face enormous time pressures. Nursing education has become more sophisticated, increasing the difficulties students have with studying efficiently and keeping pace.

The need for a comprehensive, well-designed series of study aids is great, which is why we've produced Springhouse Notes...to meet that need. Springhouse Notes provide essential course material in outline form, enabling the nursing student to study more effectively, improve understanding, achieve higher test scores, and get better grades.

Key features appear throughout each book, making the information more accessible and easier to remember.

- **Learning Objectives.** These objectives precede each section in the book to help the student evaluate knowledge before and after study.
- **Key Points.** Highlighted in color throughout the book, these points provide a way to quickly review critical information. Key points may include:
  —a cardinal sign or symptom of a disorder
  —the most current or popular theory about a topic
  —a distinguishing characteristic of a disorder
  —the most important step of a process
  —a critical assessment component
  —a crucial nursing intervention
  —the most widely used or successful therapy or treatment.
- **Points to Remember.** This information, found at the end of each section, summarizes the section in capsule form.
- **Glossary.** Difficult, frequently used, or sometimes misunderstood terms are defined for the student at the end of each section.

Remember: Springhouse Notes are learning tools designed to *help* you. They are not intended for use as a primary information source. They should never substitute for class attendance, text reading, or classroom note-taking.

This book, *Community Health Nursing,* uses conceptual models, theories, concepts, and processes of community nursing as a framework for presenting the roles, functions, and practice settings in CHN. Important content areas, such as levels of prevention, epidemiology, community health financing and legislation, and organization of the U.S. health care delivery system, are also discussed. The Populations at Risk section uses a nursing process approach with specific application of CHN roles and functions across all three levels of prevention: primary, secondary, tertiary.

SECTION I

Framework for Community Health Nursing

Learning Objectives

After studying this section, the reader should be able to:

- Define community health nursing (CHN).
- Identify the distinguishing characteristics of CHN practice.
- Recognize primary care as a major CHN component.
- Define the CHN viewpoint of *health*.
- Identify key elements of CHN practice.

I. Framework for CHN

A. Characteristics of CHN practice

1. Basic concepts
   a. Focuses on preventive rather than curative care
   b. Enhances individual, family, and community group health
2. Key ideas
   a. Provides services in the context of family and community
   b. Serves clients of all ages
   c. Focuses on populations rather than individuals
   d. Collaborates with other disciplines
   e. Encourages the client's active and collaborative participation in health promotion activities
   f. Views *health* as including all degrees of illness and wellness
   g. Addresses primary, secondary, and tertiary levels of prevention

B. Elements of CHN practice

1. Promoting healthful life-style
   a. Providing health education
   b. Demonstrating healthful living skills
   c. Directing health care system efforts to provide the client with health promotion options
2. Treating disorders through direct and indirect nursing interventions
   a. Providing *direct* nursing services for sick clients, including in-home nursing care, health counseling for clients having potential or diagnosed disorders, and health education regarding illness and wellness states
   b. Providing *indirect* services that ensure assistance for clients with health problems, such as advocating new community health services, participating in resource planning and development, consulting with team members, and developing programs to correct unhealthful community conditions
3. Promoting rehabilitation
   a. Reducing client disability and restoring client function
   b. Incorporating a group focus such as ostomy clubs, Alcoholics Anonymous, or halfway houses
   c. Recognizing that increased chronic conditions in a growing elderly population have increased the need for rehabilitation
4. Providing community services
   a. Identifying community health problems
   b. Formulating community diagnoses
   c. Planning services that address community needs
5. Providing primary care services
   a. Providing health services that are the client's first contact with the health care system during any illness episode
   b. Assuming responsibility for continuum of care
   c. Providing services through the expanded role of nurse practitioner

6. Evaluating services and needs
   a. Recognizing evaluation in analyzing and improving CHN
   b. Recognizing emerging trends in health care delivery
   c. Using evaluation on the single case or program level

C. The American Nurses' Association definition of CHN

1. Basic concepts
   a. Synthesizes nursing and public health practices
   b. Strives to promote and preserve the health of populations
   c. Provides general and comprehensive care
   d. Provides continuing rather than episodic care
2. CHN focus
   a. Health promotion
   b. Health education
   c. Health maintenance
   d. Holistic management of client health care
3. CHN clients
   a. Individuals
   b. Families
   c. Groups

D. The American Public Health Association definition of CHN

1. Basic concepts
   a. Synthesizes public health sciences knowledge and professional nursing theories
   b. Seeks to improve the health of the entire community
   c. Involves multidisciplinary teams and programs
2. CHN focus
   a. Primary prevention
   b. Health promotion
   c. Identification of high-risk population subgroups
   d. Health planning
   e. Client self-help activities
3. CHN clients
   a. Individuals
   b. Families
   c. Groups

Points to Remember

CHN synthesizes public health and nursing practices.

CHN practice places a major emphasis on primary care.

The CHN viewpoint of *health* includes all degrees of illness and wellness.

Health promotion and prevention are major CHN components.

CHN clients are individuals of all ages, families, and groups.

Glossary

Continuing care—care provided over an extended time, in various settings, spanning the illness-to-wellness continuum

Continuum of care—health maintenance; symptom evaluation and management; appropriate referrals

Direct services—those involving a personal relationship with the client

Episodic care—care involving the curative and restorative aspects of nursing practice

Health—state of being that includes varying degrees of illness and wellness

Indirect services—those ensuring adequate health resources for the client

SECTION II

Historical Development of CHN Practice

Learning Objectives

After studying this section, the reader should be able to:

- Outline the historical development of CHN.
- Name prominent nursing leaders in CHN development.
- Identify significant events affecting the development of CHN education.
- Trace the evolution of modern CHN from being a home-based service to a comprehensive service in many settings.

II. Historical Development of CHN

A. Early history to A.D. 499

1. Significant nursing and health care events
   a. Earliest public health practices were sanitation measures, such as burying human excreta and removing the dead from habitation areas
   b. First therapeutic efforts were based on worship, sacrifice, and purification rituals
   c. Early Greeks understood the need for personal cleanliness, exercise, proper diet, and sanitation but ignored or destroyed the weak, sick, and crippled
   d. The Hebrew Hygienic Code (c. 1500 B.C.) established a prototype for personal and community sanitation standards, including dietary omissions and food preparation guidelines, personal cleanliness, and quarantine for individuals with communicable diseases
   e. Egyptians developed pharmaceutical preparations and constructed public drainage systems around 1000 B.C.
   f. Greeks were the first to recognize the need for trained nurses (400 to 100 B.C.)
   g. Romans made dramatic administrative and engineering advances, regulated medical practice, drained swamps, provided pure water via an aqueduct system, built sewage systems, cleaned the streets, and monitored food preparation
2. Significant CHN events
   a. Nursing care was provided by family members
   b. Romans initiated organized military nursing and built hospitals for the treatment of wounded (c. 300 B.C.)
   c. Romans developed specialized attendants for nonmilitary sick

B. 500 to 1499

1. Significant nursing and health care events
   a. Communicable disease epidemics, including cholera, leprosy, bubonic plague, and smallpox, killed millions; epidemics were caused mostly by poor personal hygiene, refuse and excreta accumulation, and poor housing conditions
   b. Community health practices disintegrated, and medical progress stopped
   c. Personal hygienic practices declined because people believed that viewing the body was immoral; people also laundered clothing infrequently
2. Significant CHN events
   a. Nurses joined military orders during the Crusades; that led to nursing care for the poor, orphaned, and sick
   b. Conventsand monasteries were used as treatment centers for the sick; several orders of nuns started providing simple nursing care to meet patients' physical needs

C. 1500 to 1699

1. Significant nursing and health care events
   a. Struggles within the Catholic church caused the deterioration of church-affiliated nursing care (c. 1500)
   b. Elizabethan Poor Law (1601) guaranteed medical and nursing care for England's blind, lame, and poor
   c. Anton van Leeuwenhoek invented the microscope (late 1600s) and observed microorganisms in soil and water
   d. Europeans began analyzing health problems and proposing solutions
   e. Hospitals became places to study and teach medicine as well as to treat the sick
   f. Leonardo da Vinci dissected the human body and recorded his findings in anatomic sketches
2. Significant CHN events
   a. Nursing care was perceived as charitable endeavor
   b. St. Vincent de Paul organized the Sisterhood of Charity in France; sisters visited the sick in their homes (1621)
   c. De Paul and Mademoiselle de Gras advocated special education for individuals helping the poor and sick; they also recognized the need for professional supervision of care providers

D. 1700 to 1799

1. Significant nursing and health care events
   a. Blockley Hospital was established in Philadelphia (1731); later became Philadelphia General Hospital
   b. Pennsylvania Hospital was founded by Benjamin Franklin and Dr. Thomas Bond (1751)
   c. The first American medical school was established in Philadelphia (1765)
   d. One of the first state hospitals for the mentally ill was founded in Williamsburg, Va. (1770)
   e. Communicable diseases were widespread in Europe; Napoleonic Wars resulted in further illness and injury among the civilian population
   f. Public health efforts suffered as the Industrial Revolution shifted the focus of cultural values and resources from quality of life issues toward industrial progress
   g. Rapid population growth coupled with a declining emphasis on health care increased infant mortality rates, unhealthful working conditions, and mental illness
   h. Edward Jenner developed the smallpox inoculation (1798)
2. Significant CHN events
   a. Hospitals, jails, and workhouses employed trained nurses, supervised by physicians, to care for the mentally ill
   b. Nursing practice lost the emphasis and prestige it held previously; nurses were recruited from lower classes and nursing practice was viewed as a lowly occupation, paralleling women's social status of the time

E. 1800 to 1899

1. Significant nursing and health care events
   a. Florence Nightingale (1820-1910) founded modern nursing
   b. England passed important public health legislation providing for sanitation measures and establishing the National Vaccination Board (1837)
   c. Edward Chadwick published the "Report on an Inquiry into the Sanitary Conditions of the Labouring Population in Great Britain" (1848); that led to the creation of a General Board of Health by concluding that health required effective sanitation, sanitation required engineering solutions, engineering and medical advisors were needed, and one authority should administer sanitation matters
   d. The "Shattuck Report" (1848) was published in Massachusetts advocating a state health department and local health boards; sanitary surveys; vital statistics record keeping; environmental sanitation; controls on food and drug production; communicable disease control measures; well-child care, including immunizations; smoke and alcohol controls; town planning; and preventive medicine instruction in medical schools
   e. Louis Pasteur confirmed the existence of airborne bacteria (1860)
   f. The American Public Health Association (APHA) was founded (1872)
   g. Linda Richards, the first American-trained nurse, graduated (1873)
   h. Nurses Associated Alumni, later renamed American Nurses' Association (ANA), was founded (1896)
2. Significant CHN events
   a. Nightingale's contributions included British military health care system reform, training schools for nurses, professional nursing standards of practice, methods for calculating mortality and other health statistics, and documenting the relationship between sanitation and disease
   b. William Rathbone, the first person to promote a visiting nurse service for the poor in Liverpool, England, personally employed a nurse to provide in-home care for the sick in the city's slums and later founded a training school for visiting nurses
   c. Organized home nursing care, called district nursing, began as a voluntary service for the poor; wealthier patients employed private nurses for home care
   d. First U.S. training schools for nurses were established (1873) at Bellevue Hospital, New York City; New Haven Hospital, Conn.; and Massachusetts General Hospital, Boston
   e. New York City Mission employed visiting nurses for the first time (1877)
   f. First district nursing associations were established in Buffalo (1885), in Boston (1886), and in Philadelphia (1886)
   g. Lay boards administered early district nursing associations and, in some cases, laypeople supervised nursing care
   h. New York City initiated district nursing service with nurse supervision (1893)

i. Lillian Wald established Henry Street Settlement House (1893) to provide services for the poor; nursing services were a major activity
j. Wald's Henry Street project marked the beginning of public health nursing; for the first time, nurses were affiliated with a board of health rather than a religious order; fees reflected the client's ability to pay; service focused on preventive and health maintenance strategies
k. Los Angeles Health Department became the first to employ a public health nurse (1898)

F. 1900 to 1970

1. Significant nursing and health care events
   a. Marie Phelan became the first nurse consultant appointed to the federal government during peacetime (1923)
   b. National League for Nursing was established (1952)
   c. Medicare and Medicaid programs were enacted (1965)
2. Significant CHN events
   a. Public health nursing expanded the district nursing focus of aiding the poor to encompass entire populations; recognized family and environmental health influences; and incorporated knowledge and skills in specialized areas such as tuberculosis, mental health, maternal-child health, and school health
   b. Public health nurses were employed by voluntary agencies, such as visiting nurse associations, and official government agencies, such as health departments; official agency affiliations grew significantly during early 1900s
   c. Lillian Wald founded school nursing; offered services of Henry Street Settlement public health nurse to the New York City school system
   d. Metropolitan Life offered first public health nursing program for policyholders (1909); program was suggested by Lillian Wald
   e. The family emerged as the unit of service
   f. National Organization of Public Health Nursing established (1912); Lillian Wald served as first president
   g. First formal CHN education offered by Teachers College in association with the Henry Street Settlement House (1914); postgraduate course taught by Mary Adelaide Nutting
   h. C.E.H. Winslow, Harry S. Mustard, and Mary Breckenridge conducted rural health demonstration projects in New York, Tennessee, and Kentucky (1920)
   i. Sheppard-Towner Act (1921) awarded grants to states willing to develop programs to assist mothers and children
   j. Estelle Massey and Mable Stauper became first black nurses invited to join the National Organization of Public Health Nurses and participate in committee work (1930)
   k. Pearl McIver, employed by the United States Health Service, became the first public health nurse to provide consultation to state health departments (1934)

l. Lucille Petry appointed Assistant Surgeon General (1949); first woman and first nurse to hold this position
m. Ruth Freeman became the first nurse appointed to the American Public Health Association executive board
n. Baccalaureate nursing programs adopted public health nursing course work in the mid-1960s
o. Medicare and Medicaid programs necessitated changes in nursing practice, including establishing home health care agencies as bases for CHN practice; revising and standardizing nursing care procedures; and expanding nursing programs to include physical therapy, occupational therapy, specialized nutrition programs, and social services
p. Innovative community programs such as neighborhood health centers, model cities programs, Volunteers in Service to America, the Peace Corps, and senior citizen centers established new public health nurse roles

G. 1971 to the present

1. Significant nursing and health care events
   a. Increased nursing political activity influenced community health service development, nursing education and research, and health policy development at the federal, state, and local levels
   b. The Center for Nursing Research was established within the Department of Health and Human Services (1985)
2. Significant CHN events
   a. CHN expanded the early public health focus by assuming care for the entire community—specifically, by adding health care of aggregates to existing responsibilities for individuals and families, developing diverse programs, providing comprehensive care by trained community health nurses, emphasizing health promotion, and serving in agencies and settings from hospitals to independent practices
   b. Growing acceptance of the disease prevention concept led to defining the role of infection-control nurse to monitor, prevent, and control hospital-acquired infections
   c. The number of public health graduate programs increased dramatically
   d. APHA adopted *public health nurse* and ANA adopted *community health nurse* as terms to describe similar nursing services, causing confusion; most nursing educators and administrators use *community health nurse*

Points to Remember

Contemporary CHN evolved from district nursing during the 1800s, to public health nursing during the early to middle 1900s, to CHN in the 1970s.

CHN started as home care for the community's poor and sick and evolved into comprehensive services, in various settings, for sick and well clients.

Lillian Wald is considered the founder of contemporary CHN.

The CHN focus has broadened from the individual to include families, groups, and entire communities.

Baccalaureate nursing programs incorporating CHN courses have created a sound educational base for CHN; the development of community and public health nursing graduate programs (including nurse practitioner programs) has advanced CHN as a nursing specialty.

Glossary

Aggregate—population group

District nursing—voluntary nursing services provided to poor and sick by charitable agencies during the 1800s; forerunners of today's visiting nurses associations

Official agency—directed and funded by a government body such as a state, county, or city

Public health nursing—expansion of district nursing to include any needy individual during the early and middle 1900s

Voluntary agency—one that relies on staff and volunteers to provide services and is funded through fees, gifts, dues, and grants

SECTION III

Conceptual Models and Theories Used in CHN

Learning Objectives

After studying this section, the reader should be able to:

- Identify the conceptual models and theories used in CHN.
- Describe the major concepts underlying each theory or model.
- Discuss the importance of each model or theory to CHN.

III. Conceptual Models and Theories Used in CHN

A. Conceptual model

1. Definitions
   a. Symbolic representation of reality
   b. Schematic representation of some relationships between phenomena
   c. Use of symbols or diagrams to represent an idea
2. Basic concepts
   a. A conceptual model attempts to describe, explain, and sometimes predict the relationship between phenomena
   b. Models are composed of abstract and general concepts and propositions
   c. Models provide organized frameworks for nursing assessment, planning, intervention, and evaluation
   d. Conceptual models facilitate communication among nurses and encourage a unified approach to practice, teaching, and research
   e. Florence Nightingale developed the first conceptual nursing model

B. Theory

1. Definitions
   a. A set of interrelated concepts providing a systematic explanatory and predictive view of a phenomenon
   b. A research-based means of interpreting phenomena in an accurate, rational, and consistent manner
2. Basic concepts
   a. Theories are logical and composed of concepts and propositions
   b. Separate theories about the same phenomenon can interrelate the same concepts, yet describe and explain them differently
   c. A theory can describe a particular phenomenon; explain relationships between phenomena; predict the effects of one phenomenon on another; and be used to produce a desired phenomenon
   d. Research performed to validate theories expands the nursing and community health body of knowledge
   e. Theories differ from conceptual models; both can describe, explain, and predict a phenomenon, but theories provide data needed to reproduce the phenomenon whereas conceptual models do not

C. Symbolic interactionism theory

1. Introduction
   a. Originated in the works of pragmatist philosophers William James, John Dewey, and George Herbert Mead
   b. Used to study and conceptualize basic social processes
   c. Applied specifically to family study by nursing and other disciplines
2. Major concepts
   a. Provides a means of understanding human interactive behavior
   b. Focuses on how individuals define their situations and on the consequences of their actions

c. Emphasizes internal family dynamics, including an individual's role definition, interactions with others, and perception of that person's role within the family
d. Analyzes how role definition and interactions develop and change over time

3. CHN implications
a. Evaluate the client, family, or community role definition and its effect on interactions
b. Work within the client's role definition
c. Assess group dynamics affecting the client
d. Help the client self-assess actions and their consequences
e. Negotiate goals for action that are mutually acceptable to the nurse and client

D. Systems theory

1. Introduction
a. Associated with the work of Ludwig von Bertalanffy
b. Provides a framework for viewing a client and his environment as an interrelated, interacting whole

2. Major concepts
a. Systems are sets of organized components that react to and interact with other systems in their environment
b. A system reacts as a whole; the dysfunction of one system component affects the entire system
c. Systems employ a feedback cycle of input, throughput, and output
d. Systems are organized in a hierarchy
e. Systems are open or closed
f. Systems have boundaries that can interact with other systems
g. A system is greater than the sum of its parts

3. CHN implications
a. Function effectively within the client system (the community) rather than the hospital system
b. Assess whether a system—individual, family, or community—is open or closed
c. Assess the system hierarchy
d. View the client as an open system that receives input from the environment and depends on interaction with the environment for growth or change
e. Evaluate whether growth within the community is positive or negative
f. Evaluate client function to identify the system's reaction to stressors
g. Use systems theory to make a complete assessment of each client within the environment
h. Use systems theory to determine, and possibly control, nursing intervention success within the client's environment

E. Developmental theory

1. Introduction
   a. Originated in 1949 during the First White House Conference on Family Life
   b. Evelyn Duvall and Reuben Hill co-chaired the conference
   c. The conference sought to summarize family problem research and document the evolution of family life
2. Major concepts
   a. Family is a social system
   b. Family is a task-performing unit
   c. Family has relatively closed boundaries
   d. Family is continually confronting and dealing with change
   e. Family development is predictable
   f. Family development should be studied comparatively, over successive generations
   g. Family development assessment concentrates on developmental tasks and role expectations
   h. Family developmental tasks occur in each family life cycle stage; each task must be completed before the family can successfully move to the next stage
3. CHN implications
   a. Apply the developmental framework to traditional and, possibly, non-traditional families
   b. Anticipate family life cycle stages and provide appropriate family guidance in the community setting
   c. Help the family anticipate developmental cycle changes and promote a clearer understanding of family roles, relationships, and responsibilities
   d. Observe the family at home to accurately assess the developmental cycle
   e. Use knowledge of developmental tasks when assessing and implementing needed community services

F. Roy Adaptation Model

1. Introduction
   a. Developed in 1970 by nurse theorist Sister Callista Roy
   b. Characterized as a systems theory with strong analysis of interactions
2. Major concepts
   a. People are adaptive systems
   b. Stimuli, or input, cause system changes
   c. System changes may be adaptive (beneficial) or maladaptive (detrimental) to the system
   d. Two mechanisms control the system: the cognator and the regulator
   e. Four modes affect or implement system adaptation: physiologic, self-concept, role function, and interdependence
3. CHN implications
   a. Use the Roy adaptation model as a framework for assessing the client and the family in the community environment

   b. Help the family achieve the optimum state of adaptation by manipulating stressful stimuli
   c. Try to maintain and maximize family modes of adaptation
   d. Help the family change maladaptive behavior to adaptive behavior
   e. Develop a comprehensive plan of care by assessing the four adaptive modes
   f. Use the Roy adaptation model as a basis for client education and health promotion planning

G. Rogers' Science of Unitary Man

1. Introduction
   a. Developed in 1970 by nurse theorist Martha Rogers
   b. Based on general systems theory
   c. Includes developmental model elements
2. Major concepts
   a. Individuals and their environments are viewed as energy fields characterized by wave patterns
   b. Individuals are open systems, interacting continuously with the environment; a state known as openness
   c. Systems exhibit pattern and organization
   d. Systems have four-dimensionality
3. CHN implications
   a. Use Rogers' Science of Unitary Man to promote and maintain health, prevent disease, and diagnose and intervene in illnesses
   b. Provide client care in all settings and actively plan to provide future care in settings such as space stations and moon colonies
   c. Help the client achieve optimum health potential
   d. Promote a harmonious interaction between the client and the environment
   e. Direct and redirect client system and environment patterns and organization

H. Johnson's Behavior Systems Model

1. Introduction
   a. Developed in 1968 by nurse theorist Dorothy Johnson
   b. Based on systems theory
   c. Includes behavior model subsystems
2. Major concepts
   a. Behavior system contains seven subsystems: affiliation, achievement, aggression, dependence, elimination, ingestion, and sexual
   b. Subsystems have four elements: drive or goal, predisposition to act, action alternatives, and action or behavior
   c. Entire behavior system, including subsystems, has functional requirements of protection, nurturing, and stimulation

3. CHN implications
   a. Promote the efficient and effective health-related behavior in human systems
   b. Analyze the seven subsystems of a client's behavior as functional or dysfunctional
   c. Use four modes of intervention: limiting behavior, providing protection from negative stressors, suppressing ineffective responses, and providing nurturing and stimulation
   d. Help the client change ineffective responses to effective responses in the home environment

I. Orem's Self-Care Model

1. Introduction
   a. Developed in 1959 by nurse theorist Dorothea Orem
   b. Characterized as a systems model and an interaction model
   c. Evolved from Orem's view that nursing should promote self-care
2. Major concepts
   a. Self-care denotes performing personal activities necessary to maintain life, health, and well-being
   b. Self-care requisites are categorized as universal, developmental, and health deviation
   c. Self-care agency refers to a person's ability to perform self-care actions
   d. Dependent care agency refers to a person's ability to provide care for an individual unable to perform self-care
   e. Therapeutic self-care demand is the composite of self-care actions necessary to maintain an individual's health
   f. A self-care deficit occurs when therapeutic self-care demand exceeds self-care agency
3. CHN implications
   a. Implement nursing systems that are wholly compensatory, partially compensatory, or supportive-educative
   b. Use these systems to meet the self-care needs of an individual, family, or community until self-care agency is restored
   c. Help the client learn self-care skills that promote optimum health in the home or community setting
   d. Examine universal, developmental, and health deviation self-care requisites when assessing community health needs
   e. Use this assessment when planning community health services and programs
   f. Help the client assume responsibility for personal health needs
   g. Teach the family how to promote lifelong self-care

J. Neuman's Systems Model

1. Introduction
    a. Developed in 1972 by nurse theorist Betty Neuman
    b. Characterized as an open systems model with two components: stress and stress reaction
    c. Based on Gestalt theory and psychology field theories
2. Major concepts
    a. Individual is depicted by concentric circles with impacting stressors
    b. The core, or center, of the circles represents those things necessary for life
    c. The outer circle represents the flexible line of defense against stressors
    d. The middle circle represents the normal line of defense
    e. The third circle, protecting the inner core, represents lines of resistance
    f. Stressors are characterized as intrapersonal, interpersonal, and extrapersonal
3. CHN implications
    a. Promote stability in the client and the client system within the environment
    b. Assess the client's and nurse's stressor perceptions
    c. Organize assessments into psychosocial relationship categories, physical status, developmental characteristics, and spiritual influences
    d. Keep in mind that the nursing goal is to protect the core structure
    e. Intervene to prevent stressor impact during primary prevention, reduce the impact of stressors in secondary prevention, and restore optimal client function through tertiary prevention

K. King's Theory of Goal Attainment

1. Introduction
    a. Developed in 1968 by nurse theorist Imogene King
    b. Characterized as a systems theory and an interaction theory
2. Major concepts
    a. Individuals are social, sentient, rational, reactive, perceptive, controlling, purposeful, action oriented, and time oriented
    b. Individuals have three subsystems: personal, interpersonal, and social
    c. The personal subsystem encompasses perception, self, growth and development, body image, space, and time
    d. The interpersonal subsystem encompasses human interaction, communication, transaction, role, and stress
    e. The social subsystem encompasses organization, authority, power, status, and decision making
    f. Effective transactions or communication between client and nurse promote satisfaction and ultimately goal attainment
3. CHN implications
    a. Assess the client's personal, interpersonal, and social subsystems to identify attainable goals
    b. Work with the client to establish goals for optimum health

c. Promote meaningful transactions between the client and the environment
d. Develop a goal-oriented nursing record for individuals, families, and communities

L. Maslow's Theory of Hierarchy of Needs

1. Introduction
   a. Developed in 1949 by Abraham Maslow
   b. Proposes that human behavior is motivated by needs that are arranged hierarchically from basic to complex
2. Major concepts
   a. Motives influence behavior
   b. Motivation is internal and results from individual feelings and needs
   c. Basic needs must be met before higher-level needs
3. CHN implications
   a. Assess the client and environment to determine the level of hierarchical need
   b. Develop a plan of care based on the client's current level of need
   c. Create a climate of motivation by helping the client meet current level of needs
   d. Prioritize plan of care to the client's level of need
   e. Use Maslow's hierarchy when assessing community needs and developing community services

Points to Remember

Conceptual models and theories are necessary guides for nursing practice.

Theories and models are derived from nursing practice and other disciplines.

Both theories and conceptual models can describe, explain, or predict relationships between phenomena; however, only theories present the information needed to reproduce a phenomenon.

Because of the scope of CHN practice, community health nurses have opportunities to use models and theories with different client populations, in different settings.

Glossary

Adaptation—ability to change in response to a stressor

Cognator—human subsystem control mechanism responsible for logical and rational thought processes

Partially compensatory system of nursing assistance—nurse and client share responsibility for meeting therapeutic self-care demands

Regulator—human subsystem control mechanism responsible for adapting responses to stressors

Supportive-educative system of nursing assistance—client requires only education and social support to meet the therapeutic self-care demand effectively

Wholly compensatory system of nursing assistance—nurse is responsible for meeting all client therapeutic self-care demands

SECTION IV

Concepts Used in CHN

Learning Objectives

After studying this section, the reader should be able to:

- Identify concepts used in CHN.
- Discuss each concept's importance within CHN.
- Identify the three levels of prevention and their CHN applications.

IV. Concepts Used in CHN

A. Levels of prevention

1. General information
   a. First described in 1953 by H. R. Leavell and E. G. Clark, who identified primary, secondary, and tertiary approaches to preventive medicine
   b. Gerald Caplan described three levels of prevention for psychiatric medicine in the 1960s
   c. Levels of prevention overlap; roles and functions of the community health nurse at each level are not always clear; functions for one level of prevention may apply to other levels
2. Key ideas
   a. *Primary prevention*: intervening in the natural progression of a disease before pathologic changes occur in the client; involves health promotion and specific protection—for example, immunization; reduces incidence of disorders by preventing their occurrence
   b. *Secondary prevention*: detecting and treating a disease early, which decreases the duration of the disorder and limits disability
   c. *Tertiary prevention*: limiting disability or restoring function; includes rehabilitation
3. CHN implications
   a. Incorporate the three levels of prevention into practice, thereby serving individuals, groups, and communities in all stages of illness and wellness
   b. Direct health promotion efforts to enhance the general well-being of the individual, family, or community
   c. Engage in specific protection activities, including immunizations, health counseling, and safety measure enforcement in the home, school, workplace, or other community setting
   d. Provide health counseling on subjects such as nutrition, exercise, and stress management to promote healthful life-styles
   e. Participate in early diagnosis and treatment by making effective assessments and referrals and by performing selected screenings and examinations
   f. Help limit disability by referring clients with known but untreated disorders; participating in a hospice program; counseling clients with advanced disease states or chronic disorders about their need for treatment; and referring clients having chronic diseases, but lacking effective treatment, to appropriate resources and services
   g. Participate in activities that assist rehabilitation, such as recommending exercises as part of a rehabilitation program for a client or participating in community organizations and programs that serve disabled and handicapped clients

LEVELS OF APPLICATION OF PREVENTIVE MEASURES

The chart below, developed by H.R. Leavell and E.G. Clark, shows the natural history of a disease as it relates to the three levels of prevention, then identifies specific activities that can be used for each level of prevention.

NATURAL HISTORY OF A DISEASE

Prepathogenesis period	Pathogenesis period
Interrelations among Agent, Host, and Environmental Factors → Stimulus	Early Pathogenesis → Discernible Early Lesions → Advanced Disease → Convalescence

LEVELS OF PREVENTION

Primary prevention		Secondary prevention		Tertiary Prevention
Health promotion	*Specific protection*	*Early diagnosis and prompt treatment*	*Disability limitation*	*Rehabilitation*
Health education Good standard of nutrition adjusted to developmental phases of life Attention to personality development Provision of adequate housing, recreation, and agreeable working conditions Marriage counseling and sex education Genetics Periodic selective examinations	Use of specific immunizations Attention to personal hygiene Use of environmental sanitation Protection against occupational hazards Use of specific nutrients Protection from carcinogens Avoidance of allergens	Case-finding measures, individual and mass Screening surveys Selective examinations Cure and prevention of disease processes Prevention of the spread of communicable diseases Prevention of complications and sequelae Shortened period of disability	Adequate treatment to arrest disease process and prevent further complications and sequelae Provision of facilities to limit disability and prevent death	Provision of hospital and community facilities for retraining and education for maximum use of remaining capacities Education of the public and industry to employ the rehabilitated As full employment as possible Selective placement Work therapy in hospitals Use of sheltered colony

Adapted from Leavell, H.R., and Clark, E.G. *Preventive Medicine for the Doctor in His Community,* 3rd ed. New York: McGraw-Hill Book Co., 1965.

B. Epidemiology

1. General information
   a. First studied by Hippocrates (460-377 B.C.) as he tried to explain disease occurrence on a rational rather than supernatural basis—specifically, that environment and life-style are related to disease occurrence
   b. Most early epidemiologic investigations focused on infectious disease occurrence
   c. Epidemiologic investigation techniques were first developed in the mid-1800s when infectious diseases ravaged Europe
   d. John Snow studied factors associated with cholera outbreaks in England during the 1850s and associated mortality rates in specific regions with sources of contaminated water
   e. Nursing epidemiology originated with Florence Nightingale's detailed description of military conditions in the Crimea, an early and systematic descriptive study of the distribution and pattern of disease in a population
   f. Current epidemiologic investigations focus on infectious disease; noninfectious chronic conditions such as heart disease, cancer, and stroke; acute events such as accidents; emotional and mental disorders; and characteristics of normal and well populations
2. Key ideas
   a. Disease occurs when an *agent* is present in a susceptible *host* under *environmental* conditions favorable to pathogenesis; these interrelationships are used to study a disease's history
   b. Patterns of health or illness in populations are assumed to result from the interaction of many forces; known as *multiple causation*
   c. The primary epidemiologic measurement is rate, the number of times that a disease or condition occurs in a population during a specific period
   d. Descriptive epidemiology studies health problem incidence and prevalence within a population
   e. Descriptive epidemiologic processes can identify populations at risk for developing health problems
   f. Primary, secondary, and tertiary levels of prevention can be used for identified risk populations
   g. Analytic epidemiology identifies variations in incidence or prevalence by studying health problem determinants
   h. Analytic epidemiology employs four types of studies: cross-sectional, retrospective, prospective, and experimental
   i. A cross-sectional study selects a population and observes for the condition or event at one time; yields prevalence data
   j. A retrospective study selects two groups of people—one with a specific condition such as an illness, the other free of the condition (control group); historic data are gathered and studied to determine whether exposure to certain factors can be associated with the condition's development

COMMON EPIDEMIOLOGIC RATES

MORTALITY

$$\text{Crude mortality rate} = \frac{\text{Number of deaths within a given time}}{\text{Midyear population}}$$

(expressed per 1,000, 10,000, or 100,000 of population)

$$\text{Specific mortality rate} = \frac{\text{Number of yearly deaths for a specified group}}{\text{Mean yearly population for the group}}$$

(expressed per 1,000 of population)

$$\text{Maternal mortality rate} = \frac{\text{Number of deaths from pueperal causes in a year}}{\text{Number of live births in that same year}}$$

(expressed per 100,000 live births)

$$\text{Infant mortality rate} = \frac{\text{Number of deaths of children under age 1 in a year}}{\text{Number of live births in that same year}}$$

(expressed per 1,000 live births)

MORBIDITY

(expressed per 1,000, 10,000, or 100,000 of population)

$$\text{Incidence} = \frac{\text{Number of new cases of disease in a place from time}_1\text{ to time}_2}{\text{Population at midpoint of time}_1\text{ to time}_2}$$

$$\text{Prevalence} = \frac{\text{Number of cases in a place at a given time}}{\text{Population in a place at the same time}}$$

k. A prospective study follows a group of people through time to chronicle condition or event onset; yields incidence data
l. An experimental study manipulates variables; one group is exposed to a specific factor and a control group is not; both groups are studied over time to chronicle condition or event onset
m. Epidemiologic investigation information sources include vital statistics records, census data, reportable disease registries, environmental monitoring agencies, and the National Center for Health Statistics and Health Survey
n. Epidemiology can be used to study the effects of disease and wellness states in populations over time and predict future health needs, diagnose community health, evaluate health services, estimate a client's risk according to group experience, identify syndromes, complete the clinical picture so that prevention measures can be taken before a disease becomes irreversible, and search for a disease's cause

3. CHN implications
   a. Understand the agent-host-environment relationships (web of causation) that produce multiple causation of disease in individuals, families, and communities

b. Understand and use incidence and prevalence rates to summarize health data frequencies
c. Use epidemiologic data to identify health problem risk factors
d. Use epidemiologic data to identify high-risk populations
e. Use epidemiologic data to determine which risk factors can reduce a specific health problem
f. Use epidemiologic data to plan programs that meet individual, family, and community health needs
g. Establish program priorities by diagnosing the community's current state of health and describing changing community health problems
h. Use epidemiologic methods similar to the nursing process when planning community and aggregate care
i. Institute prevention and control measures based on epidemiologic information

C. Program planning and evaluation

1. General information
   a. American Public Health Association (APHA) emphasized the need for better program planning by public health officers as early as the 1920s
   b. In 1944, the American Hospital Association initiated regional health service planning
   c. Congress passed the Hill-Burton Act, an early piece of health planning legislation, in 1946
   d. The Community Health Centers Act of 1963 gave states the authority to plan mental health programs
   e. The Regional Medical Program Act of 1965 encouraged joint health care study through planning groups comprised of health care providers and consumers
   f. The National Health Planning and Resources Development Act of 1974 specified the structure, process, and functions of a national health planning system and created a health systems agency (HSA) for each service area to develop a health systems plan and annual implementation plan; plans were reviewed by a statewide health coordinating council
   g. Sharp federal funding cuts beginning in 1980 prompted many states to assume responsibility for HSAs; in 1981, states either established their own health systems or dismantled existing health systems along federally mandated guidelines
   h. In 1982, federal funds were allocated to continue HSA closings; currently, no federal, state, and consumer health partnership exists
2. Key ideas
   a. The five phases of the health care planning process are the preplanning phase of stating the goal, delineating a timetable, assessing resources, and defining data collection strategies; the assessment phase of assessing needs, setting priorities, and specifying objectives; the policy

development phase of assessing strategies for achieving objectives and negotiating needed organizational liaisons; the implemention phase; and the evaluation phase

b. Program planning defines what the organization and health care provider are attempting to do for the client

c. Assessing the need for a program is the most important step in health program planning

d. An assessment of need employs census data, key informants, community forums, surveys of agencies and residents, statistical indicators, and risk estimates

e. Planning methods include five key approaches and models: *Planning, Programming, and Budgeting System*—an outcome-oriented accounting system used by agencies to determine efficient resource allocation; *Program Planning Method*—a five-stage process involving clients, providers, and administrators to determine needs and solutions; *Program Evaluation Review Technique*—a programming method for large-scale projects that uses concepts of time and events to plan, schedule, and control numerous activities; *Critical Path Method*—a programming method that focuses on critical (vital) activities, sequence, and duration and identifies needed resources; and *Multi-Attribute Utility Technique*—a planning method based on decision theory

f. Planning for evaluation is integral to the planning process; evaluation is often omitted unless it is clearly identified as an integral program component

g. Evaluations may be conducted to determine a program's relevance, progress, efficiency, effectiveness, or impact

h. The Structure-Process-Outcome model, developed by Avedis Donabedian, is a widely used evaluation model

3. CHN implications

a. Use clinical practice experience to identify consumer concerns and service gaps or duplications

b. Take part in the health planning process for population groups by participating in health planning teams and providing valuable input that accurately reflects the holistic needs of the population group

c. Contribute to the evaluation of program relevance and progress; contrast program participant needs with program components

d. Analyze family needs in addition to population needs; provide input on clients' perceived needs

D. Quality assurance

1. General information

a. Present-day community health and CHN quality assurance activities are based on the efforts of early nursing and public health leaders

b. During the 1860s, Florence Nightingale pioneered efforts to set standards of care, advocated a uniform format for collecting and presenting hospital statistics to identify and correct hospital treatment deficiencies, and established the foundation for contemporary quality assurance activities used in CHN

c. Between 1912 and 1939, concern about the quality of nursing education led to nursing program accreditation by qualified organizations; accreditation resulted in higher nursing education standards; CHN benefited as well-educated, better-prepared community health nurses entered the field
d. Nursing licensure was required in all states by 1923; all nurses were required to meet uniform standards of preparation for practice
e. Post-World War II nursing focused on developing a scientific method for nursing practice; later evolved into the nursing process, a systematic approach to nursing and CHN
f. The Phaneuf Nursing Audit, developed in 1952, has been used extensively in CHN practice; used in home health agencies as a peer review mechanism
g. Problem-Oriented Medical Record System was established by Lawrence Weid in 1969 to assure documentation of health care evaluations
h. Professional Standard Review Organizations were established in 1972 to ensure the effective and economic use of Medicare, Medicaid, and other federal funds
i. CHN practice standards were established in 1973 and revised in 1986; CHN quality care criteria were established; community health nurses are responsible for maintaining these standards
j. Professional Review Organizations (PROs) were established in 1983 to monitor the prospective reimbursement system based on diagnosis-related groups (DRGs) for Medicare recipients
k. Definitions of CHN by the American Nurses' Association (ANA) and APHA strengthened CHN practice

2. Key ideas
   a. Evaluation is the nursing process component that addresses quality assurance
   b. Quality assurance uses general and specific approaches
   c. General approaches include licensure, accreditation, and certification
   d. Specific approaches include staff and peer reviews, the audit process, utilization reviews, PROs, evaluation studies, client satisfaction assessments, and performance appraisals
   e. The audit process is an important tool that helps peer review committees determine the quality of care provided
   f. The six audit process steps are selecting the study topic, selecting explicit quality care criteria, reviewing records to determine if the criteria were met, conducting a peer review in cases where quality care criteria were not met, recommending specific actions to correct the deficiency, and following up to ensure that the problem is eliminated

g. Audits may be concurrent, evaluating the quality of ongoing care, or retrospective, evaluating the quality of care after client discharge
h. Utilization review may be prospective, concurrent, or retrospective
i. Utilization review assures that care is needed and that cost is appropriate for the level of care provided
j. The ANA has developed a quality assurance program model

3. CHN implications
   a. Serve on the health care team monitoring the quality of client and community services provided by the agency
   b. Participate in peer reviews and the agency audit process
   c. Demonstrate a concern for the quality of care at all levels of CHN practice—individual, family, and community

E. Change theory

1. General information
   a. In 1951, Kurt Lewin applied concepts from field theory to the process of change
   b. In 1976, Robert Chin and Kenneth Benne proposed three strategies for implementing change: empirical-rational, normative-reeducative, and power-coercion
2. Key ideas
   a. Change is constant and inevitable
   b. Planned change is conscious, deliberate, and collaborative
   c. The goal of change is improved operation of the human systems
   d. The nurse's role as change agent is based on change theory
   e. According to Kurt Lewin, field theory forms the foundation of contemporary change theory
   f. Field theory stages include unfreezing, a dissatisfaction with the present system; moving, implementation of the change; and refreezing, the practice of a newly acquired behavior until it is stable
   g. Change theory applies to changes in individuals as well as organizations
3. CHN implications
   a. Identify factors affecting the unfreezing process, such as the presence and sources of dissatisfaction
   b. Promote refreezing after change has occurred by role modeling newly established behaviors and supporting the client's adoption of new behavior
   c. Use change theory principles when planning and effecting changes in the community
   d. Use change theory for planning changes in organizations
   e. Use change theory as a base for effective management

F. Leadership theories and models

1. General information
   a. Early researchers fell into one of two groups concerning leadership qualities: those who believed that individuals were born with leadership qualities, and those who believed individuals acquired leadership qualities
   b. Some early theories proposed that one factor determined effective leadership—for example, the great person theory, trait theory, situation theory, or interaction theory
   c. Recent studies have focused on leadership behaviors instead of personality traits as the definitive factors in determining leadership effectiveness
2. Key ideas
   a. Leadership is the process of influencing individual or group activities in relation to a goal
   b. Leadership is composed of styles or theories
   c. Leadership styles are autocratic, democratic, and laissez-faire, which refer to the leader's control in relation to the freedom available to subordinates
   d. The Tri-Dimensional Leader Effectiveness Model, a widely accepted leadership model that proposes leadership skills can be taught and learned, was developed in 1977 by Paul Hersey and Kenneth Blanchard; the model proposes that leaders choose a leadership style appropriate for the situation; the leader considers task behavior, relationship behavior, and subordinate maturity when selecting appropriate leadership style
3. CHN implications
   a. Provide leadership in various situations involving other community health professionals
   b. Evaluate the current situation, the task or goal to be accomplished, the needs of the group as a whole, and individual and relationship needs within the group
   c. Promote quality care by providing effective leadership
   d. Serve as a leader in life-style management and health promotion by demonstrating positive health behaviors, such as eating nutritious foods, exercising regularly, maintaining normal weight, not smoking, and effectively managing stress
   e. Use leadership principles in many areas of practice, education, supervision, and administration
   f. Use leadership principles whether or not a leadership title is possessed
   g. Use leadership principles to promote effective group dynamics in families and the community

SECTION V

Processes Used in CHN

Learning Objectives

After studying this section, the reader should be able to:

- Describe the processes employed to improve community health.

- Discuss the scope and diversity of the processes used to promote health.

- Discuss the importance of each process to CHN.

Points to Remember

Levels of prevention can be used to describe any component of CHN practice.

The community health nurse uses epidemiology to identify high-risk groups, aggregates, or populations and to design programs to alleviate the health problem.

Assessing the needs of the group or population is the most basic component of program planning and should be conducted carefully to ensure that the need is accurately identified.

Change theory helps the community health nurse understand the organizations in which she works and her role in the change process.

The community health nurse can effectively use leadership principles whether or not she is identified as the leader.

Glossary

Agent—factor whose presence or absence causes disease

Environment—all external conditions and influences

Epidemiology—study of the distribution and determinants of health, health conditions, and disease in human populations

Host—human being that provides an environment for disease

Incidence—rate of newly occurring cases of a disease in a population during a specific period

Natural history of a disease—process by which a disease occurs and progresses, involving the interaction of agent, host, and environment

Prevalence—number of existing cases of a disease in a defined population at a given time

Risk—probability of an unfavorable event, such as developing a disease

V. Processes Used in CHN

A. The helping relationship

1. General information
   a. Defined as a purposeful interaction between the nurse and client involving mutual participation
   b. Seeks to benefit the client by meeting specific client health needs; differs from social relationships that address the needs of each relationship participant; the nurse's needs are not addressed in the helping relationship
2. Key ideas
   a. Exists to benefit the client rather than the nurse
   b. Involves an explicit mutual agreement that specifies what the relationship will involve
   c. Assigns responsibilities to the client and nurse
   d. Sets beginning and ending relationship boundaries
   e. Requires skilled communication by the nurse
   f. Involves three phases: initiating, working, and terminating. In the initiating phase, the nurse and client introduce themselves; the nurse explains her role and establishes a verbal contract stipulating the location, frequency, and length of meetings as well as overall relationship purpose and method for handling confidential information. In the working phase, the nurse identifies the client's needs, formulates and implements a care plan, and evaluates the work after interventions are completed. In the terminating phase, the relationship ends; successful termination is signified by nurse and client ambivalence; can induce a sense of loss of a meaningful relationship
   g. Requires planning for termination during initiating phase; relationship evolves as the nurse and client focus on the reasons each is involved in the relationship
3. CHN implications
   a. Use the helping relationship for successful interactions with individuals, families, and groups in the community setting
   b. Initiate the helping relationship within the community setting where the client often has a greater sense of self-confidence
   c. Use the helping relationship to carry out all aspects of nursing practice
   d. Use the helping relationship to facilitate primary prevention in the client's home before illness or hospitalization are needed
   e. Use the helping relationship when assisting clients with necessary secondary and tertiary prevention measures

B. Contracting

1. General information
   a. Defined as a systematic method of increasing desirable client behavior
   b. Characterized by continuous and negotiable flexibility based on mutual understanding and trust

c. Used in the helping relationship
d. Helps the client develop self-care abilities by requiring that he perform specific, desirable health behaviors

2. Key ideas
a. Client and nurse partnership requires mutual agreement and participation
b. Client and nurse commit to fulfilling the contract's purpose
c. Terms of the partnership, such as purpose, respective responsibilities, and limits, are defined
d. Necessary contract modifications are achieved through negotiations
e. Effective client contracts include written, realistic, measurable goals; clearly stated target dates; and rewards for goal accomplishment
f. Both parties retain a signed, dated copy of the contract

3. CHN implications
a. Use contracting when promoting client self-care in the home or community setting
b. Assess the client's daily environment and then work with the client to establish reasonable goals
c. Use contracting to improve a client's problem-solving skills
d. Assist and instruct the client, family, and other significant individuals before contract initiation
e. Use contracting in primary prevention to help a client eliminate a health risk, such as smoking
f. Use contracting in secondary prevention to increase the client's compliance with prescribed treatment regimens in home and community settings
g. Use contracting in tertiary prevention to promote client adherence to life-style changes necessitated by illness, or adherence to long-range treatment programs, such as those for I.V. drug abusers or recovering alcoholics

C. Crisis intervention

1. General information
a. A crisis is a temporary state of severe disequilibrium felt by individuals facing a situation they find threatening; they can neither escape the situation nor resolve it with existing problem-solving skills
b. Crisis intervention, based on crisis theory, is the systematic application of problem-solving techniques
c. Crisis intervention moves the client through the crisis as quickly and painlessly as possible and restores the client's psychological comfort to a level equal at least to the precrisis level
d. Crisis theory was developed by Gerald Caplan in 1961 and was augmented by Eric Lindemann's work in 1979

2. Key ideas
a. Crisis is a temporary condition, with disequilibrium lasting 4 to 6 weeks
b. Reactions to crisis can be predicted and may be prevented

   c. Developmental crises occur in response to the stress in predictable life transitions and events
   d. Situational crises occur when unanticipated events threaten an individual's biological, social, or psychological integrity
   e. Social crises occur when uncommon events—for example, fires or earthquakes—cause multiple losses or severe environmental changes
   f. Crisis involves cognitive uncertainty, not understanding the situation and not knowing its outcome
   g. Crisis evokes psychological and physiologic symptoms
   h. Crisis results when an individual's coping process proves ineffective or insufficient, causing severe disorganization
   i. Individuals in crisis experience disorganization and heightened stress levels and may exhibit exaggerated defense mechanisms and feelings of helplessness
   j. Individuals in crisis are healthy people temporarily unable to cope effectively
   k. Crisis increases an individual's vulnerability to illness and, concurrently, presents the individual with an opportunity to grow into a healthier state
   l. Crisis precipitation and resolution is related to the perception of the event or situation as realistic or unrealistic, the availability of support systems, and the client's coping mechanisms

3. CHN implications
   a. Focus only on the crisis event and related issues when implementing the nursing process
   b. Use a supportive approach to crisis resolution by providing the client with a means of expressing feelings in the nonthreatening environment of the home or community setting
   c. Employ an educative approach to help the client understand new events and apply this information in the familiar home and community settings
   d. Teach problem-solving skills based on identified strengths and weaknesses in the client's environment
   e. Focus on restoring the client to a state of equilibrium in his environment
   f. Facilitate an open expression of client feelings and emotions as part of the home or community assessment

D. Stress management

1. General information
   a. An early stress theory focusing on the physiologic stress response was proposed by Hans Seyle during the 1950s; Richard Lazarus proposed another theory in 1966 that focused on the psychological stress response
   b. Stress results from physical or psychological forces that require an individual to alter his coping modes
   c. Stress is directly and indirectly related to many physical and emotional illnesses

2. Key ideas
   a. Stress develops when an individual appraises a situation and finds that the demand for change exceeds his ability to cope
   b. Stress increases when an individual faces personal, social, and environmental changes
   c. An individual's stress is based on his perception of a situation as neutral, benign, or stressful
   d. How an individual experiences stress depends on an event's predictability and social context, the individual's degree of control over the situation, and the individual's coping skills
   e. Tolerable stress can motivate an individual toward goal achievement
   f. Stress indicators include physical, behavioral, and emotional factors
   g. Stressors are internal or external stimuli that trigger physiologic and psychological coping mechanisms
   h. Stressors can elicit a physiologic response, as described by Seyle's General Adaptation Syndrome, or a psychological response
   i. Stress can be managed by altering an individual's exposure to the stressor, environment, or perception of the stressor
   j. Stress management techniques include muscle relaxation, meditation, creative imagery, hypnosis, exercise, biofeedback, acupressure, and therapeutic touch
   k. Support from reliable and caring groups, such as family, friends, and work associates, is valuable when coping with stress
3. CHN implications
   a. Inform the client that everyone experiences stress and that stress can be managed effectively
   b. Teach stress management strategies to individuals, families, and groups in the community setting
   c. Use stress management during primary prevention with individuals, families, and groups experiencing a stressful situation
   d. Help parents become effective role models and stress management skills teachers in their homes
   e. Serve as a role model for the client by implementing a personal stress reduction program

E. Health education

1. General information
   a. Health education has been a key CHN component since the days of Florence Nightingale and Lillian Wald
   b. Health education is based on learning theories, including stimulus-response, cognitive-discovery, and humanistic
   c. *Stimulus-response* learning theories developed by Ivan Pavlov, John Watson, Edward Thorndyke, and B.F. Skinner posit that students learn in a structured, systematic manner, with stimuli planned to arouse specific responses

   d. *Cognitive-discovery* learning theories developed by Jean Piaget, Max Wethmeimer, and Kurt Lewin focus on the individual's tendency to establish a stable and coherent perception of the world and to experience the world as a meaningful whole
   e. *Humanistic* learning theories developed by Abraham Maslow, Carl Rogers, and Arthur Combs emphasize the importance of emotions, values, attitudes, and self-expression
   f. The PRECEDE (Predisposing, Reinforcing, and Enabling Causes in Education Diagnosis and Evaluation) model of health education proposes that multiple factors produce health and health behavior; health education must be multidimensional and influence health behavior within the context of home and community
   g. The Health Belief Model of health education states that individuals will not adopt preventive behaviors unless they possess a minimum level of relevant knowledge and motivation, believe they are vulnerable to health disruptions, view the disruptive condition as threatening, are convinced of the usefulness of intervention, and envision few difficulties in proceeding with the recommended actions
2. Key ideas
   a. The three learning domains are cognitive, affective, and psychomotor
   b. The cognitive domain deals with recall, or knowledge recognition
   c. The affective domain describes changes in interests, attitudes, and values
   d. The psychomotor domain includes observable performance of skills that require some degree of neuromuscular coordination
   e. Successful education programs are based on teaching and learning principles
3. CHN implications
   a. Teach clients of all ages, in all phases of illness and wellness, keeping in mind the client's environment and health status and available community resources
   b. Use education in primary prevention to reduce risk factors in the home, workplace, and community settings
   c. Use education in secondary prevention to inform the client about early signs and symptoms of illness and available treatment resources
   d. Promote tertiary prevention by teaching necessary life-style modifications and health protection strategies
   e. Assess the client's environment carefully to develop a teaching plan appropriate for the client's situation
   f. Design effective teaching strategies by assessing the cognitive abilities of the client and significant others to target the most appropriate learner
   g. Consider the specific needs of adult learners
   h. Evaluate the effectiveness of all teaching

F. Health promotion

1. General information
   a. Care that promotes health and prevents illness, when possible, is more desirable than an approach that treats an illness after it occurs
   b. Activities that promote healthful life-styles have the potential for increasing longevity, improving the quality of life, and reducing health care costs
   c. Health promotion is the central component of primary prevention
2. Key ideas
   a. Health promotion is creative self-fulfillment; an actualization of inherent and acquired potential
   b. Health promotion differs from disease prevention by not only seeking to limit disease but maximizing an individual's potential in all facets of life
   c. A family that values health is likely to engage in health-promoting behaviors
3. CHN implications
   a. Use anticipatory guidance and education as the primary health promotion activities with individuals, families, and community groups
   b. Assess the client's health-promoting behavior to identify barriers to new behavior implementation
   c. Plan health promotion approaches with the client to fit his value structure and goals
   d. Teach the client about health promotion activity and guide him to resources needed to adopt the activity
   e. Support the client's efforts to adopt the recommended health promotion behavior
   f. Evaluate with the client the process of incorporating the behavior into his life-style; discuss making modifications as needed

G. Continuity of care

1. General information
   a. Assesses, plans for, and meets the client's ongoing health needs
   b. Promotes smooth client transitions from one level of care to the next
   c. Requires client and family participation and multidisciplinary planning
   d. Contains two integral components: discharge planning and referral process
2. Key ideas
   a. Discharge planning is the development, implementation, and evaluation of a design for the continuity of care of a client who will terminate his relationship with a health care provider
   b. Effective discharge planning assures that the client's health care needs will be met as he moves to the next level of care

c. Discharge planning concentrates on matching client and family needs with community resources and on helping the client and family adapt to the changing situation
d. Discharge planning relies on the involvement of the family and significant others
e. Referral is the systematic problem-solving process that helps the client use available home and community resources to meet his needs
f. The referral process includes an assessment of client referral needs, the selection of resources, the referral, and an evaluation of the referral

3. CHN implications
   a. Begin discharge planning early in the health care process
   b. Consider client and family needs within the context of existing family dynamics and relevant physical, psychosocial, and environmental factors
   c. Use the community service referral process to help the client effectively meet his health care needs
   d. Respond promptly to a referral by visiting the client or by phoning within 24 hours
   e. Collaborate with other health team members to establish and continue discharge planning services in the community

Points to Remember

The helping relationship is the basis for all intervention processes.

Health education, always an important part of the community health nurse's role, continues to be the primary intervention strategy for improving client self-care and health-promoting activities.

The community health nurse uses stress management and crisis intervention to maintain or restore a client's state.

Discharge planning and referrals are two integral components of continuity of care.

Glossary

Crisis—temporary state of disequilibrium experienced by an individual lacking the coping skills needed to address a situation he deems threatening and inescapable

Health education—combination of learning experiences designed to facilitate voluntary behavior adaptations conducive to health

Health promotion—individual and community activities that increase the level of well-being and actualize the potential of individuals, families, and community groups

Learning—change in behavior that persists over time; may be positive or negative and may result in growth

Teaching—communication process employed to change the learner's behavior

SECTION VI

Roles and Functions of Community Health Nurses

Learning Objectives

After studying this section, the reader should be able to:

- Identify factors influencing CHN roles.
- Describe the community health nurse's care provider role.
- Discuss the health educator role.
- Identify role model functions.
- List the important advocate role characteristics.
- Describe four modes of counselor intervention.
- Discuss the researcher role functions.
- Contrast the manager, leader, and consultant roles.

VI. Roles and Functions of Community Health Nurses

A. Introduction

1. CHN incorporates various roles that the community health nurse uses in many settings
2. Roles may blend or overlap
3. The community health nurse must be flexible, adapting to client needs and situations
4. Underlying all community health nurse roles is letting the client function independently to promote self-reliance
5. Factors influencing roles include:
    a. Organization or agency policy
    b. Community sociocultural norms
    c. Public perception of CHN
    d. Legal guidelines and restrictions
    e. The nurse's personal values and norms
    f. The nurse's perception of each role's requirements
    g. The nurse's adaptability to changes in community health care needs

B. Care provider role

1. Basic concepts
    a. Clients are individuals, families, or groups
    b. CHN care is holistic, involving the client's physical, psychological, social, and spiritual needs
    c. The community health nurse provides care to clients across the health continuum
    d. Care is comprehensive, encompassing primary, secondary, and tertiary levels of prevention
2. Functions
    a. Provide *direct* care to sick clients in various settings, assessing client needs and formulating a plan of care that includes bathing, range-of-motion exercises, medication, treatments, ambulation, and environment adaptation
    b. Provide *indirect* care to sick clients in various settings, discussing the illness and care requirements with the client and family members, coordinating nursing care with other health care providers, explaining services available from other community agencies, and referring clients to appropriate community resources
    c. Guide the health maintenance and promotion activities of all clients by assessing individual health practices, encouraging clients to consider the importance of their health, recommending health practice changes when needed, and supporting family strengths and positive health practices
    d. Provide care appropriate to each level of prevention

C. Health educator role

1. Basic concepts
   a. Teaching is the foundation of health education: it addresses topics relevant to all client health stages and all levels of prevention
   b. Health education lets the client assume more responsibility for meeting his own health needs
   c. Health education may involve individuals, families, or community groups
   d. Of all health care providers, community health nurses are the best suited to provide health education because of their holistic health care approach and understanding of family dynamics
   e. Community health nurses realize that the family plays a significant role in the client's learning and that information learned by the client affects the entire family
   f. Health education promotes better daily health practices, enhances the client's coping skills, and provides strategies for dealing with specific health problems
2. Functions
   a. Assess the client's need for instruction by determining what the client knows, needs to know, and wants to know
   b. Provide a well client with primary prevention and health promotion through health education
   c. Provide health education to a client recovering from illnesses on such subjects as medication, hygiene, treatments, ambulation, and signs and symptoms of complications; instruction may be formal, informal, or both
   d. Arrange community health education programs on health and wellness topics such as nutrition, exercise, stress management, diseases and disease management, and effective treatments
   e. Teach information relevant to the client's health and life-style; topics range from specific information concerning an illness, such as administering medication, to general information about life-styles or developmental stages, such as retirement leisure time planning.
   f. Help the client select appropriate sources of health information from books, magazines, television, friends, and relatives

D. Role model

1. Basic concepts
   a. A role model is someone whose behavior is adopted by others
   b. A role model illustrates specific behavior patterns
   c. As a role model, the community health nurse gives each client an opportunity to observe positive health practices and effective problem-solving strategies
   d. The community health nurse's actions communicate valuable health information
   e. Clients are individuals, families, and groups
   f. Role modeling is used in primary, secondary, and tertiary levels of prevention

2. Functions
   a. Demonstrate positive physical and mental health practices, such as eating nutritious foods, maintaining desirable weight, exercising regularly, not smoking, arranging time to relax daily, and communicating effectively
   b. Maintain a professional appearance, conveying that similar standards apply to work
   c. Approach problems and make decisions in a calm, thoughtful, and rational manner using systematic, effective problem-solving skills
   d. Illustrate the uses of problem-solving skills in everyday situations

E. Advocate role

1. Basic concepts
   a. An advocate actively represents the legitimate needs of another
   b. CHN advocacy seeks to foster client independence and improve the health care system so that it responds to client needs
   c. An effective advocate is assertive, willing to take risks, and able to communicate clearly, negotiate thoroughly and convincingly, and identify and tap resources for the client's benefit
   d. Advocacy is practiced for all clients—individuals, families, and community groups
   e. Advocacy is used in primary, secondary, and tertiary levels of prevention
2. Functions
   a. Arrange services for the client who is unable to do so
   b. Communicate with referral agencies to facilitate the client's transition from one agency to another
   c. Participate in community planning efforts that promote the development of client health resources
   d. Help develop policies within an agency or organization to ensure that client health needs will be met
   e. Point out inadequate or unjust services
   f. When appropriate, coordinate health care team efforts and participate in the care delivered by the team
   g. Collaborate with health team members
   h. Facilitate continuity of care among care providers by using clear and concise verbal and written communications
   i. Help the client make optimal use of health care resources
   j. Improve the client's access to health care resources
   k. Help fellow health care professionals recognize and plan for individual, family, group, and community health needs
   l. Promote client advocacy in all agency activities

F. Counselor role

1. Basic concepts
   a. The goal of counseling is effective problem solving
   b. Effective counseling is based on a positive and helping relationship

   c. Counseling can involve individuals or families, may involve a group (such as a support group), and may take place in the home, clinic, or other setting
   d. Counseling can be used in primary, secondary, and tertiary levels of prevention
2. Functions
   a. Provide information, listen objectively, and be supportive, caring, and trustworthy
   b. Help the client identify the problem and relevant factors
   c. Guide the client as he explores approaches to the problem and choices for solving the problem
   d. Promote clear thinking by helping the client avoid irrelevant distractions
   e. Help the client find a workable solution to the problem

G. Manager role

1. Basic concepts
   a. A manager uses specific skills to coordinate the activities of others to achieve a specific goal
   b. Some manager roles require advanced education
   c. Clients served by the manager include individuals, families, and community groups
   d. Effective management helps the community health nurse meet goals for primary, secondary, and tertiary levels of prevention
2. Functions
   a. Supervise client care
   b. Supervise ancillary health team members, such as home health aides
   c. Manage larger systems of clients and employees, such as a home care agency or outpatient clinic
   d. Coordinate agency and community planning activities

H. Researcher role

1. Basic concepts
   a. The researcher role focuses on investigation, a responsibility of all nurses
   b. Effective research requires a spirit of inquiry, an open mind, careful observations, and systematic analysis of information and situations
   c. Certain situations require researchers with advanced education
   d. Beneficiaries of the community health nurse's research include individuals, families, groups, and communities
   e. Research is used to investigate topics in primary, secondary, and tertiary levels of prevention
2. Functions
   a. Appraise nursing, public health, and health care research, incorporating relevant concepts into practice
   b. Use established criteria when evaluating studies
   c. Read and critique research reports regularly

   d. Participate in the research of others, such as epidemiologists, health planners, and other nurses
   e. If appropriate, design and implement studies using the steps of the research process

I. Consultant role

1. Basic concepts
   a. A consultant provides professional advice, services, or information to a client intending to help solve a specific problem or improve the client's skills; some situations or tasks require advanced education
   b. Consultation is a voluntary, temporary process of interaction or communication involving two or more individuals
   c. CHN consultation seeks to encourage more self-care responsibility in the client, help the client interact constructively with others, and help the client internalize flexible and creative skills
   d. Consultation employs four intervention modes: catalytic, confrontation, prescriptive, and theory and principles
   e. The community health nurse may function as an internal or external consultant
   f. The internal community health nurse consultant is a full-time employee of an organization—a generalist or specialist hired as a facilitator and resource
   g. The external community health nurse consultant provides contract services to organizations other than an employer and serves as a facilitator and resource for a specified time
   h. Clients retaining internal and external community health nurse consultants may be groups, organizations, and communities; individuals and families are better served by less structured consulting relationships
   i. Consultation may be used in primary, secondary, and tertiary levels of prevention
2. Functions
   a. Consult with co-workers about methods for improving care and enhancing continuity of care
   b. Consult with agencies contracting for services, such as a school district, and provide problem-solving and program development guidance
   c. Consult with individuals and families about health promotion
   d. Provide guidance with learning skills or health program development when consulting with community groups

J. Leadership role

1. Basic concepts
   a. Leadership is the exercise of influence over the actions of others to accomplish a specific goal
   b. CHN clients served by this community health nurse role include individuals, families, and community groups

   c. The community health nurse uses leadership to accomplish goals in primary, secondary, and tertiary levels of prevention
2. Functions
   a. Influence the decision-making process of clients and co-workers
   b. Stimulate health promotion interest by building practice on all three levels of prevention
   c. Share relevant health promotion information with clients and colleagues
   d. Support health promotion organizations and programs
   e. Initiate therapy appropriately with individual and family clients
   f. Manage the caseload efficiently and effectively
   g. Contribute ideas for agency program development
   h. Communicate the need for health promotion policies and programs to agency officials
   i. Support policy-influencing groups such as the American Nurses' Association (ANA) and the American Public Health Association
   j. Participate in policy formation by holding elected or appointed offices in health-related organizations
   k. Influence professional changes by adhering to the ANA standards of CHN practice and effectively carrying out CHN roles

ANA STANDARDS OF COMMUNITY HEALTH NURSING PRACTICE

Standard I	Theory: The nurse applies theoretical concepts as a basis for decisions in practice.
Standard II	Data collection: The nurse systematically collects data that are comprehensive and accurate.
Standard III	Diagnosis: The nurse analyzes data collected about the community, family, and individual to determine diagnoses.
Standard IV	Planning: At each level of prevention, the nurse develops plans that specify nursing actions unique to client needs.
Standard V	Intervention: The nurse, guided by the plan, intervenes to promote, maintain, or restore health, to prevent illness, and to effect rehabilitation.
Standard VI	Evaluation: The nurse evaluates responses of the community, family, and individual to interventions in order to determine progress toward goal achievement and to revise the data base, diagnoses, and plan.
Standard VII	Quality assurance and professional development: The nurse participates in peer review and other means of evaluation to assure quality of nursing practice; the nurse assumes responsibility for professional development and contributes to the professional growth of others.
Standard VIII	Interdisciplinary collaboration: The nurse collaborates with other health care providers, professionals, and community representatives in assessing, planning, implementing, and evaluating programs for community health.
Standard IX	Research: The nurse contributes to theory and practice in community health nursing through research.

From American Nurses' Association: Standards of community health nursing practice, Kansas City, Mo., 1986. Reprinted with the permission of ANA.

Points to Remember

Community health nurses frequently assume different roles simultaneously.

Manager and leadership roles are complementary.

The advocacy role is incorporated into all CHN roles.

All roles address the primary, secondary, and tertiary levels of prevention.

Glossary

Catalytic mode of intervention—consulting that clarifies existing data or provides additional information

Collaboration—health care providers working as a team

Confrontation mode of intervention—consulting tactic of presenting information that illustrates a client's true values and assumptions

Consultation—process of helping the client perceive, understand, and act on events in the environment

Coordination—conscious effort to assemble and direct the efforts of a group of health care providers

Prescriptive mode of intervention—consultant explicitly tells the client how to solve a problem

Research—systematic investigation of phenomena

Theory and principle mode of intervention—consultant teaches the client relevant theories and illustrates their use in problem solving

SECTION VII

Practice Settings in CHN

Learning Objectives

After studying this section, the reader should be able to:

- Identify CHN practice settings.
- Describe CHN roles and functions for each setting.
- Discuss the CHN implications for each practice setting.
- Identify the program components for CHN practice settings.

VII. Practice Settings in CHN

A. Introduction

1. CHN practice settings vary greatly
2. In all settings, the community health nurse may deliver services addressing primary, secondary, or tertiary levels of prevention
3. In many settings, CHN practice places special emphasis on health promotion programs
4. The community health nurse may assume numerous roles in a given practice setting; roles may be assumed simultaneously
5. Changes in the health care delivery system require flexibility by the community health nurse in the roles and functions performed in all practice settings

B. Home setting

1. Basic concepts
   a. The home has always been the traditional setting for CHN services
   b. CHN views individuals as components of the family unit
   c. Family dynamics are readily apparent in the home setting
   d. Environmental factors that affect the family's health are observable in the home setting
2. Types of home care
   a. *Home health care:* an arrangement of health services provided in the client's home; focuses on ill-client services and incorporates a multidisciplinary health team that includes nursing services, physical therapy, speech therapy, occupational therapy, nutritional guidance, home health aide services, and social services; services may be provided by official, voluntary, or proprietary agencies
   b. *Hospice care:* a palliative system of health care for terminally ill clients and their families; services can be delivered in the client's home or in an institution, such as a free-standing clinic or hospital-based unit, and focus on improving the client's quality of life, not life extension, with an emphasis on providing comfort by controlling pain and other symptoms; may include home health services, financial assistance, respite care, chaplain support, and bereavement support for the family after the client's death
3. CHN roles in the home setting
   a. Care provider
   b. Counselor
   c. Health educator
   d. Advocate
   e. Manager
4. Functions of the *care provider* in the home setting
   a. Develop comprehensive plans of care that consider the physical, psychological, social, and spiritual needs of the family unit and include an assessment of the functioning family system

   b. Observe and evaluate the client's physical and mental condition
   c. Provide direct care—administering treatments, assisting with range-of-motion and rehabilitation exercises, administering medications, inserting catheters, irrigating colostomies, and caring for wounds
   d. Help the client and family members develop effective coping behaviors
   e. Involve family members in client care
   f. Identify the health needs of clients in health stages across the health continuum
   g. Guide and support the family in the care of an ill family member
   h. Guide the health maintenance and promotion activities of all family members
5. Functions of the *counselor* in the home setting
   a. Assist in family problem solving
   b. Help family members consider various solutions to determine which will best meet the family's needs
   c. Promote effective family communication to enhance problem solving
   d. Communicate that the family is responsible for choosing a solution alternative
6. Functions of the *health educator* in the home setting
   a. Develop formal and informal teaching programs as the situation dictates
   b. Select teaching methods and materials appropriate for the family's needs and interests
   c. Teach family members the skills and strategies needed to care for the ill family member
   d. Suggest ways for family members to incorporate newly learned health practices into the family's life-style
   e. Instruct families in health maintenance and promotion and focus on such life-style behaviors as nutrition, exercise, and stress management
7. Functions of the *advocate* in the home setting
   a. Demonstrate effective communication techniques for the home setting
   b. Select and arrange client services
   c. Collaborate with other health team members involved with the client
   d. Point out inadequate or unjust services while working to develop health care services that address community needs for home care
8. Functions of the *manager* in the home setting
   a. Manage comprehensive care for individuals and families
   b. Coordinate multidisciplinary health team activities in home and hospice care
9. CHN implications for the home setting
   a. Provide primary health care
   b. Understand that the routine health care delivery situation is reversed in the home setting where the community health nurse is a "guest" and the client feels comfortable and secure and is often more receptive to instruction
   c. Promote family strengths, family unity, and family developmental tasks by working with individuals and the entire family in various nursing roles

d. Emphasize the family's self-care responsibilities
e. Help all individuals in the family become as independent as their abilities, skills, and interests allow

C. School setting

1. Basic concepts
   a. Community health nurses first entered the school setting during the early 1900s in response to the growing problem of childhood communicable diseases
   b. The community health nurse in the school setting is usually referred to as the *school nurse*
   c. The school health program usually consists of three components: health services, health education, and environmental health and safety
   d. The school nurse collaborates with school personnel to develop and implement a health program that covers the three program components
   e. The school health program promotes optimal student health, enhancing each student's learning potential
   f. School nurses work in public and private preschools, elementary and secondary schools, and colleges
   g. School-age children health concerns include acute and chronic illnesses, accidents, abuse and neglect, drug abuse, and developmental disabilities
   h. Adolescent health concerns include acute and chronic illnesses, accidents, abuse and neglect, alcohol and drug abuse, suicide prevention, adaptation to physical and psychological development changes, teenage parenthood and sexuality, and adaptation to role changes during child-to-adult role evolution
   i. College population health concerns vary greatly because of the wide age range of students attending college
2. CHN roles in the school setting
   a. Care provider
   b. Health educator
   c. Counselor
   d. Advocate
   e. Manager
   f. Consultant
   g. Leader
   h. Role model
3. Functions of the *care provider* in the school setting
   a. Treat minor student illnesses and injuries
   b. Treat emergency conditions and arrange for appropriate medical care
   c. Assess student health concerns, providing appropriate care
   d. Conduct screening tests of vision, hearing, height and weight, scoliosis, blood pressure, and dental health to identify health problems
   e. Provide direct services, such as screenings and health guidance, to school personnel, according to school policy

   f. Conduct physical examinations, if a nurse practitioner
   g. Identify students with health needs and make referrals for appropriate follow-up (case-finding)
4. Functions of the *health educator* in the school setting
   a. Instruct students and teachers, individually and in groups, in health maintenance and promotion topics
   b. Arrange teaching programs for students on topical subjects, including nutrition, developmental changes, sexuality, first aid, and dental care
   c. Develop curricula for school health instruction programs
   d. Conduct staff education sessions to discuss current information about relevant health issues and to inform the staff about illness and injury policies and procedures
5. Functions of the *counselor* in the school setting
   a. Listen objectively, inform, and provide support to students in the problem-solving process
   b. Make necessary referrals to others, such as the guidance counselor or mental health professional
   c. Provide students with problem-solving counseling on relevant issues, such as drug and alcohol use or sexuality
   d. Clarify the nurse's role with the guidance staff to preclude conflicts and promote continuity of care
6. Functions of the *advocate* in the school setting
   a. Represent student health needs to teachers, administrators, and parents
   b. Communicate relevant information about students to teachers and administrators
   c. Identify student health program needs and inform school officials of program and funding requirements
   d. Identify high-risk student populations and develop program objectives to meet their needs
   e. Facilitate comprehensive community health care planning and resource development that address the health needs of students and their families
7. Functions of the *manager* in the school setting
   a. Maintain student health records
   b. Develop student health programs
   c. Involve other school personnel in student care when necessary
   d. Discuss a student's chronic health condition, such as diabetes, with the student's teacher and school staff when necessary
8. Functions of the *consultant* in the school setting
   a. Consult with parents on the health concerns of their children
   b. Consult with school personnel on health-related matters
   c. Recommend policies and procedures that promote school health program goals
   d. Consult with community groups on school-age population health needs
   e. Represent the school health program to community groups
   f. Participate in school planning for the educational needs of handicapped and exceptional children

9. Functions of the *leader* in the school setting
   a. Direct school health efforts in the school and community
   b. Participate in community groups that influence student health
   c. Serve as an elected or appointed member of relevant community groups
   d. Represent the health needs of students and their families when participating in communitywide health care and resource planning
   e. Participate in organizations that influence student health, such as the American Nurses' Association (ANA), the American Public Health Association (APHA), and the School Health Association
10. Functions of the *role model* in the school setting
    a. Demonstrate through daily activities positive health practices, such as exercising regularly, eating nutritious foods, not smoking, and managing stress effectively so that students and the school staff can observe desirable health behaviors
    b. Apply effective problem-solving techniques daily to illustrate positive coping behavior for students and staff
11. CHN implications for the school setting
    a. Realize the potential for delivering health services to a major population segment
    b. Positively influence future student health practices
    c. Influence school health program development, an important component in a complete student education
    d. Promote an overall improvement in school health by working to reduce absenteeism and increase learning and social productivity

D. The workplace setting

1. Basic concepts
   a. A person's job is a major health influence; work-related injuries and illnesses can cause major health status alterations
   b. The workplace is a good location for health service delivery because most healthy adults work
   c. A person's job has a significant effect on the family
   d. Workers may be exposed to biological, chemical, mechanical, physical, and psychosocial health hazards
   e. Leading work-related diseases and injuries in the United States include occupational lung disease, musculoskeletal injuries, occupational cancers, severe occupational traumatic injuries, cardiovascular disease, reproductive disorders, neurotoxic disorders, noise-induced loss of hearing, dermatologic conditions, and psychological disorders
   f. Worker safety is the major emphasis of occupational health; the Occupational Safety and Health Act of 1970 mandated comprehensive occupational safety and health programs
   g. Occupational health programs range from worker safety and illness and injury prevention to health promotion and primary prevention services
   h. Health promotion is becoming widely recognized as a legitimate and valuable facet of occupational health programs

   i. Occupational health care is an interdisciplinary team effort that may involve nurses, physicians, safety experts, counselors, addiction counselors, nutritionists, exercise physiologists, and health educators
   j. The community health nurse practicing in the workplace is often called an *occupational health nurse*; some settings now require nurse practitioner services
   k. Community health nurses practice in the following workplace settings: factories, offices, stores, hospitals, and other health care facilities
2. CHN roles in the workplace setting
   a. Care provider
   b. Health educator
   c. Counselor
   d. Advocate
   e. Manager
   f. Consultant
   g. Leader
   h. Role model
3. Functions of the *care provider* in the workplace setting
   a. Treat minor illnesses and injuries in the workplace
   b. Treat emergency conditions and refer clients as necessary for appropriate medical care
   c. Identify high-risk populations and conduct screening tests to discover such health problems as vision abnormalities, hearing impairment, and high blood pressure
   d. Guide healthy clients toward health-promoting behaviors, such as eating nutritious foods, exercising, and managing stress effectively
   e. Establish and maintain a safe work environment that is conducive to positive physical and mental health
4. Functions of the *health educator* in the workplace setting
   a. Teach relevant concepts, such as nutrition, exercise, stress management, and not smoking to healthy individuals and groups
   b. Instruct workers in accident prevention and safety promotion
   c. Instruct workers with health problems in the management of their illnesses or disabilities to maximize their ability to function
   d. Develop workplace health programs that emphasize wellness to promote healthful worker life-styles
   e. Provide health education to community groups outside the workplace
5. Functions of the *counselor* in the workplace setting
   a. Counsel workers to facilitate problem solving
   b. Refer workers and their families to other counseling resources, such as an in-house counseling staff or outside agency, when necessary

6. Functions of the *advocate* in the workplace setting
   a. Represent employee health needs to management
   b. Promote policies, procedures, and programs that optimize employee health
7. Functions of the *manager* in the workplace setting
   a. Prepare an annual budget proposal of funding needed to support nursing services
   b. Manage all aspects of the nursing services provided in the workplace setting
8. Functions of the *consultant* in the workplace setting
   a. Consult with management on health and safety issues
   b. Inform management of the health needs and concerns of the employees and high-risk populations in the work force
9. Functions of the *leader* in the workplace setting
   a. Promote positive health and safety practices in all aspects of employee relations
   b. Participate in organizations that promote employee health, such as the ANA, the APHA, and the American Association of Occupational Health Nurses
10. Functions of the *role model* in the workplace setting
   a. Demonstrate healthful practices in daily activities, such as eating nutritious foods, exercising regularly, not smoking, and managing stress effectively
   b. Wear appropriate safety clothing while in the workplace
11. CHN implications for the workplace setting
   a. Positively influence the health of a significant portion of the adult population through practice in the workplace setting
   b. Develop an awareness of working women's health issues as more women enter the work force
   c. Consider ways to encourage family unity and strength in work force families

E. Ambulatory care settings

1. Basic concepts
   a. Ambulatory care begins when a client requests health care from a qualified provider in the community
   b. Ambulatory care focuses on primary care
   c. Ambulatory care settings may be hospital or community based; examples include ambulatory care units, clinics, neighborhood health centers, centers such as medical care walk-in centers, cardiac rehabilitation programs, mental health centers, and community outreach locations
   d. Community-based services may be provided in conjunction with a larger service program, such as a senior citizens center or an adult day-care center

   e. Neighborhood health centers provide services to a geographically defined population; centers are located in urban and rural areas and may be free-standing buildings, storefronts, church basements, or mobile units
   f. Some ambulatory care centers serve specific high-risk populations, such as children, elderly people, Native Americans, migrant workers, or people living in remote areas
   g. Nurse practitioners who are primary care specialists may deliver specific ambulatory care services; areas of specialization include family health, adult health, pediatric care, family planning, gerontology, and nurse midwifery
   h. Primary care services may take place in institutional residences, such as correctional facilities, nursing homes, halfway houses, drug treatment centers, group homes for the mentally retarded or for recovering mentally ill patients, and camps
2. CHN roles in ambulatory care settings
   a. Care provider
   b. Health educator
   c. Manager
   d. Advocate
3. Functions of the *care provider* in ambulatory care settings
   a. Provide direct, comprehensive services to ambulatory individuals and families
   b. Treat clients with acute or chronic illnesses
   c. Administer care to sick and well clients
   d. Perform intake screening
   e. Treat emergency conditions and refer clients as necessary for appropriate medical care
   f. Guide individual and family health promotion and maintenance activities
4. Functions of the *health educator* in ambulatory care settings
   a. Provide formal and informal health promotion and maintenance education programs
   b. Develop educational programs that promote client self-care
   c. Present health promotion and maintenance education programs to community groups
5. Functions of the *manager* in ambulatory care settings
   a. Manage ambulatory care facility nursing services
   b. Manage client caseload
   c. Distribute client caseload to appropriate team members
   d. Supervise other health team members
6. Functions of the *advocate* in ambulatory care settings
   a. Represent target population needs to the community
   b. Guide clients to needed services within the health care delivery system

   c. Support health care legislation and initiatives that promote the development of high-quality, comprehensive ambulatory care facilities and services
   d. Support professional organization efforts to develop nurse practitioner networks in order to expand services
7. CHN implications for ambulatory care settings
   a. Realize that the demand for CHN services in cost-effective ambulatory care settings is likely to increase as health care costs rise
   b. Find expanded practice opportunities and settings as cost-effective changes occur, particularly for the nurse with advanced practitioner training
   c. Work within the community systems to increase nursing and other health service availability to community populations
   d. Work with nurse practitioners to secure third-party reimbursement for nursing services

Points to Remember

CHN practice takes place in various settings.

The home has been the traditional and prevailing setting for CHN practice.

The community health nurse focuses on the family in all practice settings.

CHN practice addresses primary, secondary, and tertiary levels of prevention in all settings.

CHN roles in ambulatory care settings have changed with the expanded role of the nurse practitioner.

Rising health care costs have expanded ambulatory care services, increasing availability, accessibility, and opportunities for CHN practice.

Community health nurses and nurse practitioners must continue to work toward third-party reimbursement for their services.

Glossary

Ambulatory care—direct personal health care services to clients seeking treatment on an outpatient, noninstitutional basis

Home health agency—voluntary, official, or private organization that provides home health care

Nurse practitioner—a post-baccalaureate health professional trained for a primary prevention role that emphasizes health maintenance and promotion and disease prevention

Primary care—accessible, comprehensive, coordinated, and continuous care provided by accountable caregivers; describes the care an individual receives during first contact with the health care system, or the continued care of the individual as an ambulatory client, or both

Private (proprietary) agency—one operated for profit

Voluntary agency—nonprofit organization supported by charity, fees, and third-party payers

SECTION VIII

Community as the Client

Learning Objectives

After studying this section, the reader should be able to:

- Define community.
- Discuss the characteristics of communities.
- Discuss the community as a unit of service.
- Describe approaches to assessing a community.

VIII. Community as the Client

A. Definitions of community

1. A group of individuals who occupy a specific geographic or governmental subdivision; for example,
   a. Residents of a city, town, or village
   b. Residents of a neighborhood within a city, town, or village
2. A group of individuals with common life-style characteristics; for example,
   a. Individuals with common interests
   b. Individuals with similar value systems
   c. Individuals with similar social systems
3. A group of individuals having a common social affiliation or concern; for example,
   a. Members of a local organization, such as the Parent-Teacher Association
   b. Members of a national organization, such as the American Nurses' Association
   c. Individuals with a common interest in a specific health issue
4. A group of individuals in which a common problem can be identified and solved; a community of need or solution; for example,
   a. A group delineated by a health or environmental problem that spans geographic or governmental boundaries
   b. A group delineated by the need to draw resources from many geographic or governmental subdivisions to solve problems effectively
5. A group of individuals comprising a locale-oriented entity; for example,
   a. An interdependent system of formal organizations that reflect social institutions, informal groups, and aggregates
   b. A group having the function or expressed intent to meet its members' common needs

B. Types of communities

1. Face-to-face community
2. Neighborhood community
3. Community of identifiable need
4. Community of problem ecology
5. Community of concern
6. Community of viability
7. Community of action capability
8. Community of political jurisdiction
9. Resource community
10. Community of solution

C. Characteristics of communities

1. A community occupies a physical space and has delineating factors, such as:
   a. Geographic or governmental boundaries
   b. Name
   c. Size and dimension

   d. System of roads and other access and exit routes
   e. Physical environment, such as housing or land use patterns
2. A community is composed of a population; criteria for identifying a population may include:
   a. Number and density
   b. Demographic structure, such as age, sex, race, and socioeconomic or geographic distribution
   c. Informal relationships
   d. Formal relationships
3. A community performs functions for its members, such as:
   a. Producing, distributing, and consuming goods and services
   b. Socializing new members
   c. Maintaining social control
   d. Adapting to changes in the surrounding environment
   e. Providing a forum for mutual aid
4. A community has assessable health characteristics that include:
   a. Vital statistics, such as birth and death rates
   b. Incidence and prevalence of leading mortality and morbidity causes
   c. Health risk profiles of selected aggregates
5. A community has a health structure that consists of:
   a. Health care facilities
   b. Health care planning groups
   c. Health care providers
   d. Patterns of health care resource use
6. A healthy community meets criteria, such as:
   a. Commitment by each member to the community
   b. Group identities and interests
   c. Effective communication among community groups
   d. Articulation by community groups of their interests and concerns
   e. Containment of conflicts
   f. Management of the community's relationships to the larger society
   g. Member participation in community activities
   h. Mechanisms for facilitating interaction and decision making among community members

D. Community as a unit of service

1. General information
   a. The community is considered the target of service when CHN practice, regardless of the setting, addresses community health concerns
   b. The community operates as a system
   c. CHN focuses on making healthful changes that benefit the whole community
2. CHN implications
   a. Identify community strengths and weaknesses, available community resources, and community population characteristics

   b. Provide care to individuals, families, or aggregates that affect the entire community
   c. Consider the community the target of service each time the community health nurse provides care
   d. Realize that a change in an individual's health affects the health of his community
   e. Know that beneficial community health changes often require concurrent changes at other social levels, ranging from personal to societal
   f. Seek healthful change with and for the community client
   g. Pursue the goal of improved community health

E. Community assessment

1. Purpose
   a. Community assessment provides the community health nurse with information that helps her know and understand the community as a target of service
   b. Community assessment identifies community health assets and liabilities
2. Types of community assessment
   a. Familiarization: assessing information about a specific individual or family as part of the community
   b. Comprehensive: assessing all information pertaining to community health
   c. Problem oriented: assessing information relevant to a specific problem
   d. Community subsystem: assessing a single aspect or dimension of community life
3. Community location assessment areas
   a. Boundaries
   b. Environment
   c. Geography
   d. Weather
   e. Environmental controls
   f. Housing
4. Community population assessment areas
   a. Age and sex
   b. Stability
   c. Education
   d. Socioeconomic status
   e. Race and ethnic background
   f. Birth, death, morbidity, and mortality rates
   g. Employment and unemployment rates
5. Community social system assessment areas
   a. Political system
   b. Education facilities and programs
   c. Recreational facilities and programs
   d. Transportation systems
   e. Employment base, such as stores, businesses, and industries
   f. Official health agencies and services

   g. Voluntary health agencies and services
   h. Health care providers
   i. Communication media
   j. Safety
   k. Relationships among community members and institutions
6. Assessment data sources
   a. Communication media
   b. Local government and community leaders
   c. Local health care agencies
   d. Libraries
   e. Churches
   f. Planning organizations
   g. Local government offices
   h. Health statistics from the local or county health department and the National Center for Health Statistics
   i. Community members
   j. Direct observations
   k. Key informants
7. Community assessment methods
   a. Survey: assessing data gathered from a representative population sample
   b. Descriptive epidemiologic study: assessing or describing health and disease phenomena in terms of time, place, and personal characteristics
   c. Participant observation: assessing a functioning social setting during direct or indirect involvment in the setting
8. CHN implications
   a. Adopt a comprehensive holistic approach to community assessment
   b. Use appropriate information sources for data collection
   c. Evaluate all aspects of the community, including its location, population, and social systems, using past and present information and, possibly, future trends
   d. Use an appropriate type and method of community assessment to achieve goals
   e. Summarize strengths and limitations relative to each assessment area
   f. When plannning interventions, consider the implications for the community and its members of each piece of information

SECTION IX

Family as the Client

Learning Objectives

After studying this section, the reader should be able to:

- Define family.
- Discuss family characteristics and functions.
- Describe family forms and types.
- Discuss the family as a CHN unit of service.
- Describe ways in which the community health nurse incorporates the concept of family as the unit of service into her practice.

Points to Remember

Community can be defined variously, but the definition always includes people, physical space, and a common purpose.

The community is the target of service when CHN practice seeks to improve community health in any setting.

Community health is the goal of CHN.

Glossary

Aggregate—population group

Community—social group determined by geographic or governmental boundaries and members who have common values and interests; composed of members who know and interact with each other through a social structure that creates and maintains norms, values, and social institutions

Key informant—one who knows the community and is willing to discuss it

Morbidity—proportion of a disease over a specified time, usually expressed as the incidence or prevalence of a disease

Mortality—proportion of all deaths occurring at a particular time and place

IX. Family as the Client

A. Definitions of family

1. Traditional: individuals united by birth, marriage, or adoption who reside together
2. Nontraditional: two or more emotionally involved individuals, from the same or different kinship groups, who comprise a household or live in close proximity and choose to identify themselves as family
3. Biological: a nuclear unit consisting of a mother, a father, and their children
4. Nonbiological
   a. Honorary relative family: a close family friend, often identified as aunt or uncle
   b. Workplace family: fellow employees or individuals in the neighborhood
   c. Chosen family: friends who are consciously or unconsciously chosen as family

B. Characteristics of family

1. A family is a social system
   a. Family members are interdependent
   b. Families set and maintain boundaries
   c. Families exhibit adaptive behavior
   d. Families exhibit goal-oriented behavior
2. A family has its shared cultural values and norms
   a. Family members have prescribed, and sometimes multiple, roles
   b. Each family has a power system
3. A family has a specific configuration, including:
   a. Nuclear family with one career
   b. Nuclear family with dual careers
   c. Reconstituted or blended family (step family)
   d. Binuclear family (joint child custody and coparenting)
   e. Nuclear dyad
   f. Single parent family
   g. Single adult family
   h. Multigenerational family
   i. Kin network
   j. Commune family
   k. Group network
   l. Unmarried single parent family
   m. Cohabiting couple, heterosexual or homosexual
   n. Cohabiting couple, heterosexual or homosexual, with children
   o. Cohabiting retired couple
   p. Institutional family, such as children in orphanages, residential schools, or correctional institutions
4. A family has structural parameters, including:
   a. Division of labor
   b. Distribution of power and authority

c. Methods of communicating
d. Boundaries
e. Relationships with other groups and systems
f. Methods of giving and receiving emotional support
g. Rituals and symbols
h. Roles

5. A family performs basic functions, including:
   a. Affective function and personality maintenance: stabilizes adult personalities and fulfills family psychological needs
   b. Socialization function: molds children into productive society members
   c. Reproduction function: produces new members
   d. Family coping function: maintains order and stability as the family interacts with its environment
   e. Economic function: provides and effectively allocates economic resources
   f. Security function: provides physical necessities, such as food, shelter, clothing, and health care
   g. Identity function: provides a sense of personal and social identity
   h. Affiliation function: provides a lifelong sense of belonging
   i. Control function: maintains order within the family and between the family and outsiders
6. A family evolves through developmental stages during its life cycle

C. Family developmental tasks

1. Beginning family
   a. Establish a marriage
   b. Relate to the kin network
   c. Plan a family
2. Early childbearing family
   a. Stabilize the family unit
   b. Reconcile family members' conflicting developmental tasks
   c. Facilitate the developmental needs of mother, father, and children (oldest child under age 2½)
3. Family with preschool children
   a. Nurture and socialize the children (oldest child between ages 2½ and 6)
   b. Maintain marriage stability
4. Family with school-age children
   a. Socialize the children (oldest child between ages 6 and 13)
   b. Promote the children's education
   c. Maintain a satisfactory marital relationship
5. Family with adolescents
   a. Balance teenage freedom and responsibility
   b. Maintain open communication between parents and children (oldest child between ages 13 and 20)
   c. Maintain marriage stability
   d. Build a foundation for future family stages

6. Launching family
   a. Release the children as they become young adults
   b. Readjust the marriage
   c. Assist aging parents
7. Middle-aged family
   a. Strengthen the marital relationship
   b. Sustain relationships with parents and children
   c. Cultivate leisure activities
8. Aging family
   a. Adjust to retirement
   b. Maintain a satisfactory home life
   c. Adjust to income changes
   d. Adjust to health changes
   e. Adjust to the death of a spouse

D. Family as a unit of service

1. General information
   a. Family is the basic social unit
   b. Family behaves as unit; effective nursing care or other therapy requires that the family be viewed as a whole
   c. Family provides support and encouragement for its members
   d. Family facilitates the physical and psychological growth of each member
   e. Family significantly influences each member's beliefs, values, attitudes, and health behavior
   f. Family fosters members' participation to effect changes
2. CHN implications
   a. Work with the family individually and collectively
   b. Begin care at the family's current, not ideal, level of function
   c. Recognize the validity of family structure variations; demonstrate an awareness of nontraditional families
   d. Emphasize family strengths
   e. Adapt nursing interventions to the family's developmental stage

E. Family health assessment

1. General information
   a. Family patterns and practices affect each member's health and the health of the family as a whole
   b. The health of each member is important to family and community health

2. Assessment areas
   a. Basic information about each family member: demographic data, personal identifying information, referral source and reason, occupation, education level, identity of significant individuals who do not reside in the household, and cultural or ethnic identity
   b. Resources available to the family: health care providers and agencies, individuals to contact in emergencies, and financial resources

c. Home environment: dwelling type and condition, safety features and hazards, adequacy of the home in meeting family needs, and changes in the home environment between visits
d. Physical and psychosocial health of each member: age, height, weight, health habits, health history, immunizations received, developmental stage, and current health status, including medications and treatments
e. Family health practices: nutrition, including food preferences, eating patterns, and special diets; recreation and leisure activities; sleep and rest patterns, including facilities and total hours of rest daily; use of health resources, including agencies and individual care providers
f. Family life-style: family values, family's relationship with the community, and attitudes toward health care

3. CHN implications
   a. Adopt a comprehensive, holistic approach to family health assessment
   b. Summarize strengths and limitations relative to each assessment category
   c. Consider the implications of each piece of information gathered about the health and functioning of family members and the family as a whole
   d. Consider all family activities that significantly relate to health assessments and that provide information for nursing diagnoses
   e. Consider the health continuum when assessing the family and make wellness-oriented diagnoses when appropriate
   f. Maintain the confidentiality of family information
4. Family health assessment tools
   a. Genogram: presents family structure and process by generation, shows health and risk factor data, and identifies members' relationships

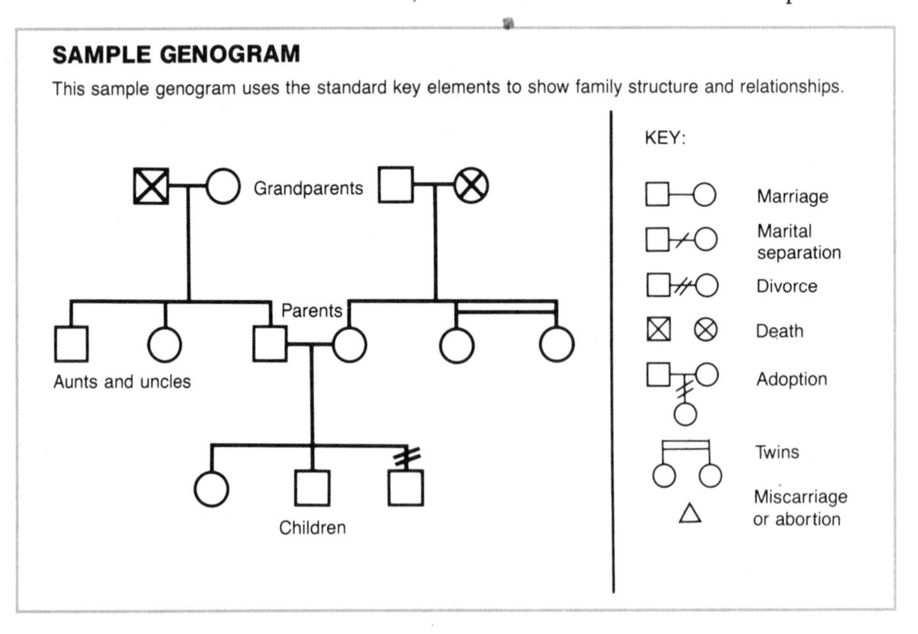

   b. Schedule of Recent Experiences Life Change Questionnaire: shows an individual the relationship between life changes and the risk of developing stress-related illness
   c. Youth Adaptation Rating Scale: measures an adolescent's ability to adapt to selected events and provides parents, teachers, and adolescents with a clearer understanding of events that may prove stressful

F. Family functioning assessment

1. General information
   a. The functioning of the family system affects each member
   b. The functioning of the family system is crucial to total family health
   c. The functioning of the family system directly affects community health
2. Assessment areas
   a. Family members' interactions
   b. Family members' developmental stages
   c. Family role relationships
   d. Family problem solving
   e. Family links with the community
   f. Family power distribution
   g. Family coping
3. CHN implications
   a. Incorporate assessment of the family system into a comprehensive, holistic assessment process
   b. Develop practice approaches that enhance family system function
   c. Emphasize family strengths to enhance family life and to improve the family's ability to cope with problems
   d. Understand that a family system assessment will take time and require ongoing contact
   e. Help family members alter family system functions by voicing observations and discussing their implications
   f. Develop strong helping relationships that involve efforts to modify the family system function
4. Family functioning assessment tools
   a. Ecomap: diagraming connections between the family system and other systems in the family's environment
   b. Family life chronology: recording family interactive processes
   c. Videotaping: directly assessing family dynamics by viewing, and reviewing, family member interactions
   d. Family sculpture: depicting each member's view of the family by arranging members in a portrait or "sculpture"; young children participate by drawing representative pictures
   e. Family coping estimate: recording the family's current coping level in 10 key areas and then estimating its ability to make changes in each area
   f. Home Observation for Measurement of the Environment: assessing the relationship between a child's home environment and development

Points to Remember

The family is the basic social unit.

Family has many definitions and is not limited to the traditional nuclear family.

Families change continuously during their life cycle.

Families have basic characteristics and structures that are expressed uniquely by each family.

The family is the basic unit of service for the community health nurse.

The health of a family member affects the entire family's health.

A family's health status affects the health of the community.

Glossary

Binuclear family—nontraditional family form composed of divorced parents sharing child custody and parenting responsibilities; children are members of two nuclear families

Commune—nontraditional family form composed of several unrelated, monogamous couples (married or unmarried) living as one household and collectively sharing child-rearing responsibilities

Dyad—two individuals, for instance a husband and wife, who maintain a significant relationship

Family developmental tasks—responsibilities in each stage of family life that must be met for family growth and preparation for subsequent tasks

Family life cycle—sequence of characteristic stages beginning with family formation, continuing through the life of the family, and ending with family dissolution

Nuclear family—traditional family unit composed of parents and their children living in one household

SECTION X

Community-Focused Nursing Practice: Populations at Risk

Learning Objectives

After studying this section, the reader should be able to:

- Identify selected populations at risk for specific physical, psychological, or social health problems.
- Identify the possible risk factors associated with specific health problems in high-risk populations.
- Identify the needs of specific high-risk populations.
- Discuss the nursing implications for primary, secondary, and tertiary levels of prevention for specific health problems.

X. Community-Focused Nursing Practice: Populations at Risk

A. Introduction

1. Populations at risk are aggregates possessing characteristics or exhibiting behaviors that increase the likelihood of developing a disease or a disorder
2. High-risk populations in a community increase demands on the health care system for services and appropriate programs, increase community health care costs, reduce community productivity, and diminish quality of life for the individual and his family
3. Health care system components responding to high-risk populations that experience chronic illnesses characterized by acute exacerbations include ambulatory care facilities, hospitals, rehabilitation centers, adult or child day-care centers, and extended care facilities
4. Heart disease and cancer account for approximately 60% of the deaths occurring in the United States each year
5. Some risk factors can be controlled or modified through nursing and public health primary prevention efforts
6. The main controllable risk factors for the leading causes of death in the United States are smoking, hypertension, elevated serum cholesterol, obesity, and alcohol and drug abuse
7. Secondary risk factors include stress and insufficient exercise; each factor is associated with several conditions and may be controllable by the individual

B. Leading causes of death in the United States

1. Cardiovascular disease
2. Cancer
3. Cerebrovascular accident (CVA)
4. Accidents
5. Chronic obstructive pulmonary disease (COPD)
6. Pneumonia and influenza
7. Diabetes mellitus
8. Suicide
9. Cirrhosis
10. Atherosclerosis

C. Clients with cardiovascular disease

1. General information
   a. Cardiovascular diseases are the major cause of death in the United States; myocardial infarction causes the most deaths
   b. Hypertensive disease is eight times more prevalent than coronary disease
   c. Death from hypertensive disease is more prevalent in blacks than whites
   d. Cerebrovascular disease is the most frequent neurologic cause of hospital admission
2. Possible cardiovascular disease risk factors
   a. Age: occurs more frequently in middle-aged and older adults
   b. Sex: occurs more frequently in males

    c. Hypertension: risk increases when blood pressure is consistently greater than 140/90
    d. Lipid abnormalities: risk increases when serum cholesterol levels are consistently greater than 260 mg/ml; triglycerides are consistently greater than 250 mg/100 ml
    e. Family history of cardiovascular disease
    f. Ethnic background: more common in blacks than whites
    g. Blood sugar abnormalities: chronically elevated blood sugar or an abnormal glucose tolerance test increases the risk
    h. Stress
    i. Obesity: increases cardiovascular disease morbidity and mortality
    j. Cigarette smoking
3. Population needs
    a. Detection and screening programs
    b. Health education to promote early detection and treatment
    c. Dietary management
    d. Medication management
    e. Restoration of optimal function by using cardiac and stroke rehabilitation programs
4. CHN functions in primary prevention of cardiovascular disease
    a. Provide family and group education on nutrition and exercise, stress management, and self-care philosophy
    b. Exemplify health promotion practices in own life
    c. Appraise the community's health for specific cardiovascular needs and problems
5. CHN functions in secondary prevention of cardiovascular disease
    a. Provide direct care to the client and family during illness episodes
    b. In community clinics, perform screening tests for elevated blood pressure and cholesterol
    c. Help the client and family adapt positively to the illness
    d. Inform client and family of available community resources
    e. Teach cardiac emergency measures
    f. Teach members of the client's family the techniques for caring for the client at home
    g. When necessary, teach the client how to monitor his own blood pressure accurately
    h. Support the development of cardiovascular health care resources within the community
    i. Support voluntary community health organizations, such as the American Heart Association
    j. Supervise ancillary personnel providing care in the client's home
6. CHN functions in tertiary prevention of cardiovascular disease
    a. Help the client perform exercises and other rehabilitation measures at home and in the community

   b. Teach the client behavior modifications, relaxation techniques, dietary modifications, and exercises to limit disability; refer to community resources when necessary
   c. Participate in community efforts to develop quality services for rehabilitation

D. Clients with cancer

1. General information
   a. Cancer is the second-leading cause of death in the United States
   b. Cancer generally occurs in all age groups, but the incidence increases with age
   c. Cancer occurs in men more often than in women
   d. Cancer mortality rates are higher for blacks than for whites
   e. Leading cancer sites in men are the lungs, prostate, and colon
   f. Leading cancer sites in women are the breasts, colon, and uterus
   g. Lung cancer is the leading cause of cancer death for men and the second-leading cause for women
2. Possible cancer risk factors
   a. Genetic background: individuals whose immediate relatives have cancer are more likely to develop a similar form of cancer
   b. Chronic exposure to chemical agents, such as asbestos, fertilizers, or coal tar
   c. Prolonged exposure to environmental agents, such as sunlight or radiation
   d. Smoking
   e. Diets high in fat or low in fiber
3. Population needs
   a. Education about possible life-style and occupational risk factors
   b. Community education about smoking hazards, including programs to help individuals wishing to stop smoking, and community education about healthful nutrition
   c. Screening tests, such as Pap smear, mammography, and stool guaiac test, to detect certain cancer types
   d. Education about early cancer signs and self-screening techniques, such as breast and testicular self-examinations
   e. Medication management
   f. Dietary management
   g. Disease management and treatment
   h. Community-based treatment and rehabilitation resources, including hospice and other support services
4. CHN functions in primary prevention of cancer
   a. Teach clients, families, and community residents how to modify high-risk life-styles
   b. Teach self-screening techniques

c. Support community efforts to discourage high-risk behaviors, such as smoking
d. Develop risk-reducing health promotion programs and resources based on epidemiologic information

5. CHN functions in secondary prevention of cancer
a. Provide direct care to the client and family in their home and community
b. Coordinate the client's use of community resources
c. Support the client and family members during disease diagnosis and treatment
d. Teach self-detection techniques to the client and family
e. Teach the client and family about necessary aspects of illness care and life-style management
f. Coordinate services given in the client's home and community
g. Supervise ancillary personnel providing care in the client's home
h. Support the development of community resources and services for risk reduction, early detection, and disease treatment
i. Participate in activities of voluntary community health organizations, such as the American Cancer Society
j. Facilitate problem solving within the family during all phases of the client's illness

6. CHN functions in tertiary prevention of cancer
a. Teach the client and family measures that facilitate the client's rehabilitation, such as dietary management, planned rest and exercise, and stress control techniques
b. Promote the development of community treatment and rehabilitation programs, including hospice programs
c. When necessary, refer the client to counseling services or other community resources

E. Clients with diabetes mellitus

1. General information
a. Between 5% and 10% of the adult diabetic population has insulin-dependent (Type I) diabetes; 80% has non-insulin-dependent (Type II or maturity onset) diabetes
b. Diabetes prevalence increases with age
c. One out of every 600 school-age children has Type I diabetes
d. Diabetes is more prevalent in women than men
e. Diabetes is more prevalent in blacks than whites
f. Diabetics experience a higher than average incidence of blindness and of kidney, vascular, and heart diseases

2. Possible diabetes risk factors
a. Family history of diabetes
b. Obesity
c. History of glucose intolerance

3. Population needs
   a. Education and resources to promote healthful nutrition and weight control
   b. Community resources for diabetes screening, early detection, and treatment
   c. Medication management
   d. Dietary management
   e. Resources, such as support groups, to teach life-style modifications necessary for diabetes control
4. CHN functions in primary prevention of diabetes
   a. Teach individuals and groups about diabetes risk factors and risk-reducing health measures, such as regular exercise, healthful nutrition, and desirable body weight
   b. Support development of community resources for wellness promotion, such as nutrition education programs and exercise facilities and programs
5. CHN functions in secondary prevention of diabetes
   a. Participate in community screening programs
   b. Refer susceptible clients for further testing and diagnosis
   c. Coordinate school efforts to assist diabetic children
   d. Provide direct care to the diabetic client and family during all illness phases
   e. Teach the client and family about diabetic care and life-style management necessary for self-care, including diet, medications, exercise, and hygiene
   f. Promote the development of treatment and resource facilities in the community
   g. Provide the client and family with community resource information
   h. Promote diabetes education for health professionals
   i. Provide client and family support during all illness phases
6. CHN functions in tertiary prevention of diabetes
   a. Instruct and support the client and family as they adapt to necessary life-style modifications
   b. Work with voluntary agencies, such as the American Diabetes Association, to promote adequate community-based treatment resources

F. Clients with COPD

1. General information
   a. COPD is the most common chronic lung disease in the United States
   b. It commonly results from an underlying condition, such as chronic bronchitis, emphysema, or asthma; underlying conditions frequently coexist
   c. COPD is a major cause of adult disability
   d. COPD occurs more frequently in men than women
   e. Approximately 75% of COPD deaths are white males
   f. COPD worsens over time

2. Possible COPD risk factors
   a. Smoking
   b. Chronic environmental or occupational exposure to high-density dusts, metals, and synthetic fibers
   c. History of recurrent or chronic respiratory infections
   d. Family history of COPD
3. Population needs
   a. Detection and screening programs
   b. Education and resources to help smokers quit
   c. Reduction of hazards to workers in high-risk settings
   d. Reduction of environmental and occupational air pollution
   e. Direct care and management of the illness
   f. Community rehabilitation programs to help individuals regain optimal function
4. CHN functions in primary prevention of COPD
   a. Teach clients and groups, especially children and adolescents, about the multiple hazards of smoking
   b. Participate in stop-smoking classes
   c. Support legislation and other measures to reduce environmental and occupational air pollution
   d. In the workplace, arrange programs to teach employers and employees about possible occupational hazards
   e. Work with management representatives to reduce airborne health hazards in the workplace
5. CHN functions in secondary prevention of COPD
   a. Provide direct care to the COPD client and family in their home and community
   b. Help the client and family adapt to changes in the client's physical capabilities
   c. Assist with community screening and detection programs
   d. Collaborate with other health care providers, including physical and respiratory therapists
   e. Teach the client and family about disease management and control measures, such as the use and care of equipment, medication, proper nutrition and hydration, and respiratory system structure and function
   f. Identify community resources for the client and family, including support groups, and facilitate their use
6. CHN functions in tertiary prevention of COPD
   a. Promote development of community-based physical rehabilitation resources
   b. Work with voluntary agencies, such as the American Lung Association, that support community-based treatment resources
   c. Teach the client and family how to adapt and modify their life-styles

G. Clients with arthritis

1. General information
   a. Arthritis is the chronic inflammation of a joint
   b. The most common arthritic disorders include rheumatoid arthritis, osteoarthritis, juvenile rheumatoid arthritis, and gout
   c. A life-crisis event may precede the onset of rheumatoid arthritis
   d. Rheumatic disease incidence and prevalence data are not routinely available
   e. A general decline of rheumatoid arthritis cases in women from 1964 to 1974 may relate to increased use of oral contraceptives
2. Possible arthritis risk factors
   a. Age: the risk of rheumatoid arthritis and osteoarthritis increases with age; gout occurs more often in middle age
   b. Sex: rheumatoid arthritis and osteoarthritis are more prevalent in women than men; gout is more prevalent in men
   c. Genetic background: purine metabolism abnormalities increase the risk of gout
   d. Joint trauma: overuse of a joint or mechanical stress on a joint increases the risk of osteoarthritis
3. Population needs
   a. Pain relief, deformity prevention, and inflammatory process control so that the client can maintain function and independence
   b. Community resources for acute and chronic disease treatment
   c. Community resources for rehabilitation
   d. Health education
   e. Medication management
   f. Research to identify causes
4. CHN functions in primary prevention of arthritis
   a. Teach correct techniques for aerobic, strengthening, and stretching exercises to well clients of all ages
   b. Promote regular, safe, and appropriate physical exercise
   c. Set up community teaching programs on arthritis risk factors for all ages; especially important for the elderly
5. CHN functions in secondary prevention of arthritis
   a. Provide direct care to the client and family in their home and community
   b. Inform the client and family of appropriate community resources, including support groups
   c. Support the client and family throughout the acute and chronic phases of the illness
   d. Teach the client and family about necessary care and life-style modifications
   e. Promote the development of community treatment and support resources
6. CHN functions in tertiary prevention of arthritis
   a. Teach the client and family how best to function within the limitations imposed by the disease

b. Encourage ongoing use of appropriate community agencies by the client and family
c. Facilitate the use of rehabilitation resources by the client and family
d. Encourage participation in community rehabilitation programs

H. Clients with sexually transmitted diseases (STDs)

1. General information
   a. The most prevalent STDs include syphilis, gonorrhea, herpes simplex, chlamydial infections, nongonococcal urethritis, and acquired immunodeficiency syndrome (AIDS)
   b. Sixteen separate STDs are currently identified by the Public Health Service and the Centers for Disease Control (CDC)
   c. Individuals with STDs commonly react with embarrassment, fear, and anger
   d. Infected individuals who engage in frequent casual sex may unknowingly infect numerous people
   e. The impact of a STD may be local or widespread
2. Possible STD risk factor: unsafe sexual practices
3. Population needs
   a. Resources for early detection and treatment
   b. Education about sexuality and STD transmission
   c. Awareness of the personal responsibility for preventing the spread of STDs
   d. Medication management
   e. Communication with the CDC
4. CHN functions in primary prevention of STDs
   a. Develop educational programs for parents and children about childhood and adolescent sexuality
   b. Develop school programs to educate children about sexuality and personal responsibility
   c. Educate individuals and community groups about STD transmission, means of prevention, and personal responsibility for preventing the spread of STDs
   d. Support programs that provide assistance to parents, children, and adolescents concerning sexuality
5. CHN functions in secondary prevention of STDs
   a. Participate in community screening and detection programs
   b. Provide direct care to the client and family during the detection, diagnosis, and treatment phases of the illness
   c. Report information to the appropriate communicable disease agency
   d. Participate in case-finding and data collection
   e. Facilitate client and family problem solving as they adapt to the implications of the disease, such as reporting contacts and life-style modifications
   f. Encourage the client to report sexual contacts

   g. Maintain case and contact confidentiality
   h. Promote development of adequate community detection and treatment resources
6. CHN functions in tertiary prevention of STDs
   a. Promote the development of accessible follow-up and referral resources for the client and family members
   b. Teach the client and family how best to function, given the limitations imposed by the disease

I. Clients with substance abuse problems

1. General information
   a. Alcohol is the most widely used substance in the United States, and approximately 10 million Americans abuse alcohol
   b. Substance *use* usually begins between ages 12 and 17, peaks between ages 18 and 34, and decreases after age 35
   c. The incidence of substance *abuse* is highest in the 18 to 25 age-group
   d. Males comprise the majority of substance abusers
   e. Since 1972, the incidence of substance abuse has risen faster for females than males
   f. Substance abuse can have devastating effects on a family
2. Possible substance abuse risk factors
   a. Family history of substance abuse
   b. Psychological or personality factors: individuals exhibiting dependency, low self-esteem, anger and frustration, depression, or omnipotent feelings have a higher-than-average risk
   c. History of other addictions
   d. Sociocultural factors: individuals needing acceptance by a sociocultural group, experiencing peer pressure, or feeling ambivalent to society have a higher-than-average risk
3. Population needs
   a. School resources and programs to educate children about substance abuse
   b. Community mental health services staffed by professionals trained in substance abuse treatment
   c. Communitywide substance abuse education, treatment, and rehabilitation efforts
   d. Support groups for substance abusers and families
4. CHN functions in primary prevention of substance abuse
   a. Teach children and adolescents about the physical, psychological, and social effects of drug and alcohol use and abuse
   b. Set up substance abuse education and prevention programs in the community
   c. Promote substance abuse education in the workplace
   d. Promote community efforts to create a drug-free environment by emphasizing the adverse effects of drug abuse
   e. Participate in and support efforts to strengthen anti-drug-use peer pressure

f. Promote development of adequate and appropriate recreational facilities for community members, especially children and adolescents
g. Promote resources that enhance mental health
h. Teach effective coping skills to clients, families, and community groups

5. CHN functions in secondary prevention of substance abuse
   a. Teach parents, teachers, children, adolescents, and others to recognize signs of substance abuse
   b. Provide direct care to the client and family during illness episodes
   c. Look for the warning signs of substance abuse—changes in appearance, hygiene, and eating habits—as part of case-finding and screening activities, particularly in school-age populations
   d. Refer clients and families to appropriate community treatment facilities, including self-help groups
   e. Help families get needed support through groups, such as Al-Anon
   f. Provide the client and family with problem-solving guidance regarding treatment
   g. Promote development of adequate, accessible community treatment facilities, especially in inner-city communities
6. CHN functions in tertiary prevention of substance abuse
   a. Promote development of high-quality, accessible rehabilitation resources and networks to assist the client and family after treatment
   b. Teach the client and family measures to promote rehabilitation and prevent problem recurrence

J. Clients experiencing violence or abuse

1. General information
   a. Half of the people murdered in the United States each year know their assailant; 30% of all murders occur within a family
   b. Family violence or abuse is difficult to detect because victims often feel guilty about the incidents or fear that filing a report will precipitate another incident
2. Possible violence or abuse risk factors
   a. Societal factors: occurs more frequently in dense population areas characterized by a high proportion of minority residents, inferior education and training facilities that foster abusive practices and disciplines, lack of community recreational facilities and social outlets, and individuals who characteristically feel powerless, helpless, or confused and lack a sense of community cohesiveness or accept or condone violence as a means to an end
   b. Family factors: incidence increases in families with autocratic and hierarchic governance, strict beliefs in corporal punishment, rigid role assignments, role reversals, social isolation, resistance to change, or a history of abusive parenting

c. Perpetrator factors: initiating violence or abuse may increase in an individual with poor self-esteem, fear and distrust of others, poor self-regulation, social isolation, lack of social skills, immature motivation toward marriage and childbearing, or poor coping skills
d. Victim factors: becoming a victim of violence or abuse may occur in an individual with learned or actual helplessness, acquired or congenital disability, poor self-esteem, social isolation, or an inability to meet spouse, caretaker, or parental expectations

3. Population needs
   a. Competent and supportive community education systems
   b. Community mental health outreach programs that support parenting and marriage relationships
   c. Social policies that promote family cohesion
   d. Treatment for victims of violence or abuse
4. CHN functions in primary prevention of violence and abuse
   a. Help the family identify problems and guide the family's use of coping and problem-solving skills
   b. Initiate and maintain a helping relationship with families at risk to promote open and trusting communication
   c. Identify a client's or family's potential for violence
   d. Anticipate family growth and development needs while providing family guidance during all family life-cycle stages
   e. Promote informed use of firearms by the general public
   f. Support community programs that promote family strengths and unity
   g. Support community efforts to provide adequate recreation and social facilities
   h. Support community efforts to provide adequate housing for low-income families
   i. Promote community efforts to provide a comprehensive network of family support services, including housing, recreation, health services, child day-care, job training, and after-school programs for children
   j. Anticipate maturational and situational family crises and counsel family members accordingly
   k. Teach positive coping behaviors to individuals, families, and community groups
5. CHN functions in secondary prevention of violence and abuse
   a. Identify signs or indicators of abuse or violence, with special attention given to vulnerable groups, such as children and elderly people
   b. Participate in programs for early detection of abuse or violence
   c. When necessary, intervene in family crises and refer one or more family members to appropriate community mental health services
   d. Provide direct care to the abused client and family
   e. Provide direct care and treatment to the abuser
   f. Develop programs to educate clients, families, and community groups about methods of dealing with violence and abuse

g. Promote development of community-based treatment programs
h. Help the family assess the need to remove a family member from the home, and then help the family plan for this possibility
6. CHN functions in tertiary prevention of violence and abuse
   a. Maintain a helping relationship with the family before, during, and after incidents of abuse or violence to maintain trust, communication, and support
   b. Coordinate nursing practice with the efforts of other health and social agencies in the community

K. Families with a pregnant adolescent

1. General information
   a. The U.S. adolescent pregnancy rate is 11% per 1,000 females and rising
   b. Currently, 1.1 million adolescent pregnancies occur each year in the United States
   c. Infants of adolescent mothers have higher rates of prematurity, low birth weight, respiratory problems, and neonatal, postnatal, and infant mortality than infants of adult mothers
   d. Pregnant adolescents experience higher rates of pregnancy complications in all categories than adult women
   e. Adolescent mothers have a high risk of social problems related to employment, interrupted education, social isolation, and role changes
2. Possible adolescent pregnancy risk factors
   a. Ignorance: inadequate understanding of sex, reproduction, and contraception increases risk
   b. Lack of contraception: inconsistent contraceptive use or difficulty in obtaining effective contraceptive methods increases risk
3. Population needs
   a. Comprehensive health and social services for mother and infant
   b. Support services that help the mother handle finances, continue her education, and plan for the future
   c. Educational resources that emphasize parenting, child growth and development, and problem-solving skills
   d. Community resources for well-baby care and follow-up
4. CHN functions in primary prevention of adolescent pregnancy
   a. Provide education to adolescents about sex and family life responsibilities
   b. Teach family planning to male and female adolescents in the home, school, and other settings
   c. Help adolescents make responsible choices and decisions about their goals
   d. Conduct outreach programs for adolescents at risk
   e. Facilitate open communication and positive relationships in the family
   f. Support efforts to make family planning services available in the schools
5. CHN functions in secondary prevention of adolescent pregnancy
   a. Deliver special prenatal and postnatal services to the mother, infant, and family

   b. Refer pregnant adolescents to sources of prenatal and postnatal care and social services
   c. Teach the adolescent family about the mother's physical and psychological health needs during and after pregnancy
   d. Teach the adolescent family how to meet the infant's physical and psychological needs responsibly
   e. Counsel the adolescent on continuing or terminating the pregnancy and make referrals to appropriate community agencies when necessary
   f. Provide counseling and emotional support to the adolescent during and after pregnancy
   g. Promote development of comprehensive, accessible community services for pregnant adolescents and their infants
6. CHN functions in tertiary prevention of adolescent pregnancy
   a. Provide direct follow-up care for the mother and infant
   b. Maintain the helping relationship as long as the adolescent needs assistance
   c. Help the adolescent avoid negative consequences of pregnancy by establishing links between the adolescent and community resources

L. Clients with mental or emotional problems

1. General information
   a. More than 15% of the U.S. population has some form of mental or emotional problem that would benefit from professional help
   b. Between 1.7 and 2.5 million individuals have chronic mental illnesses
   c. Between 0.8 and 1.5 million chronically mentally ill individuals live in U.S. communities
   d. Significant forms of mental illness include schizophrenic disorders, recurrent affective disorders, and progressive organic mental disorders
   e. Schizophrenic disorders affect 500,000 to 900,000 individuals in the United States
   f. The prevalence of chronic organic mental disorders increases with age
   g. The Community Mental Health Centers Act of 1963 established a federally assisted network of community mental health centers and mandated specific services that led to widespread deinstitutionalization of psychiatric patients
   h. Medicare and Medicaid benefits, introduced in 1965 as a means of supporting health care for elderly and indigent people, stimulated local service development
2. Possible mental and emotional problem risk factors
   a. Family history of mental or emotional illness
   b. History of inadequate coping
   c. Prolonged exposure to stress
   d. Lack of a social support system
3. Population needs
   a. Direct care and treatment for clients with mental or emotional problems
   b. Community education, treatment, and rehabilitation efforts

   c. Medication management
   d. Mental and emotional health education to promote early detection and treatment
   e. Community resources for treatment follow-up and support
4. CHN functions in primary prevention of mental and emotional problems
   a. Help the client and family develop effective coping and problem-solving skills
   b. Facilitate optimal family functioning
   c. Anticipate client crises and provide guidance as the client and family address a crisis
   d. Promote mental and physical health by teaching clients that exercise is an important aspect of stress management
   e. Advocate community development of support networks for clients and their families
5. CHN functions in secondary prevention of mental and emotional problems
   a. Participate in case-finding and intake screening
   b. Provide direct care for the client's physical and psychological functioning on a continuing basis
   c. Verify that the client swallows any prescribed psychotropic medications
   d. Help the client and family cope with mental illness and provide support as the family adjusts to the mentally ill family member
   e. Identify client signs that can indicate an impending crisis, such as discontinued medication or increased stress
   f. Identify appropriate backup services should the client become acutely ill
   g. Assist in obtaining needed client and family support, including referrals to community support groups
   h. Support development of comprehensive treatment resources in the community
   i. Participate in mental health advocacy organizations, such as the National Mental Health Association
   j. Provide educational programs on mental and emotional health for the family and community
6. CHN functions in tertiary prevention of mental and emotional problems
   a. Provide the client and family with ongoing services after the acute illness
   b. Provide support to the client and family during recovery and readjustment periods
   c. Refer the client and family to appropriate community resources, such as support groups, for follow-up
   d. Work with clients and community groups to reduce the stigma of mental illness
   e. Encourage employers to hire individuals who have received treatment for mental illness

M. Clients with AIDS

1. General information
   a. AIDS has reached epidemic proportions in the United States and has been reported in more than 40 countries worldwide

   b. By the end of 1987, approximately 50,000 AIDS cases had been reported to the CDC; the first cases were reported in 1981
   c. Projections indicate that 250,000 to 300,000 cases could be diagnosed by 1991
   d. The causative agent, human immunodeficiency virus (HIV), establishes a chronic infection that can be transmitted from person to person through specific means
   e. HIV infection can remain subclinical and unrecognized for years before causing a progressive and severe immune deficiency
   f. Projections indicate that more than 30% of HIV-infected individuals will develop AIDS 7 years after they are infected, and another 40% will develop other clinical illnesses associated with HIV infection
   g. Researchers estimate that between 1 and 2 million individuals have been infected with HIV and have antibodies to it but have remained asymptomatic during the research period
   h. Presently, data are insufficient to indicate the percentage of infected individuals who will develop AIDS
   i. Immune deficiency characteristics include numerous signs and symptoms or opportunistic infections and cancers
2. High-risk groups
   a. Homosexual and bisexual males
   b. I.V. drug abusers
   c. Hemophiliacs
   d. Individuals who received contaminated blood transfusions before donor blood screening tests
   e. Heterosexual partners of infected individuals
   f. Infants of infected mothers
3. High-risk behavior
   a. Sharing drug needles and syringes
   b. Unsafe sexual practices
4. Population needs
   a. Accessible, high-quality care in hospital settings and at home
   b. Network to provide support during the illness
   c. Acceptance by family, friends, co-workers, health care workers, and the general public
   d. Education about AIDS transmission and prevention
5. CHN functions in primary prevention of AIDS
   a. Teach members of high-risk groups about AIDS, including the disease's nature, prevention, and treatment
   b. Develop educational programs about AIDS for the general public
6. CHN functions in secondary prevention of AIDS
   a. Provide direct care to AIDS clients and families at home, carefully assessing the client's physical and psychological needs, developing a comprehensive care plan, and thoroughly executing the plan
   b. Teach infection-control measures to the client and family
   c. Support the family that provides care and comfort at home

  d. Promote a supportive home environment
  e. Advocate adequate community resources for long-term AIDS client care
  f. Support the client and family in the community
  g. Support legislation and other measures that benefit or protect AIDS patients
  h. Support measures to provide adequate funding and resources for AIDS research and treatment
  i. Help the client and family deal with AIDS treatment and implications
  j. Inform the client about AIDS support groups and other community resources as needed
7. CHN functions in tertiary prevention of AIDS
  a. Support hospice services and advocate adequate and accessible community resources for long-term care and housing
  b. Promote an understanding of AIDS and AIDS client needs in the general population
  c. Refer the client to AIDS support groups or other resources as necessary
  d. Promote the client's use of available community resources during rehabilitation and adjustment to the physical, social, and psychological aspects of the disease

N. Elderly clients

1. General information
  a. Elderly persons are individuals age 65 or older
  b. Elderly persons comprise about 11% of the U.S. population; by the year 2030, the elderly proportion will have grown to 17%
  c. The population segment over age 85 is increasing; mortality rates are decreasing more in this group than in any other population segment
  d. Most individuals over age 65 live in the community; 5% reside in institutions; 26% live alone; 22% age 85 and over live in nursing homes
  e. Chronic illnesses and health problems will increase as the elderly proportion of the population increases
  f. The major causes of illness and functional limitation in elderly clients are chronic diseases, accidents (especially traffic accidents), and stress-related conditions
  g. The most prevalent chronic conditions are musculoskeletal and orthopedic problems, heart conditions, and hypertension without heart involvement
2. Population needs
  a. Available and accessible home services for acute and chronic care, including highly technical and holistic posthospital care
  b. Medication management
  c. Coordinated services between the hospital and home
  d. Coordinated, comprehensive network of community services to maintain the independence of the elderly client and family within the health care system for as long as possible
  e. Community-based primary, secondary, and tertiary prevention services

3. CHN functions in primary prevention of disease in elderly clients
    a. Help the elderly client perform the developmental tasks of aging, such as finding adequate living quarters (at home, in a retirement community, or with children), adapting to retirement income, securing physical and emotional health protection, and feeling a personal sense of worth
    b. Counsel the elderly client regarding the life changes associated with aging
    c. Teach the elderly client about chronic disease and health problem risk factors, such as lack of exercise, smoking, excessive drinking, obesity, diets high in fat and cholesterol, environmental toxins, and accidents
    d. Provide the client with information about community resources for physical and emotional well-being
    e. Support the client's sense of self-responsibility for health
    f. Encourage participation of elderly clients and community members on citizens' councils and political action committees as spokespeople for their age-group needs
    g. Instruct the elderly client about medication schedules, therapeutic and adverse effects, and the safe use of prescribed and over-the-counter medicines
    h. Counsel the elderly client on effective and productive uses of time
    i. Support the client's family as they adapt to an aging member
    j. Counsel and educate families about the normal aging process as well as specific diseases and health problems
4. CHN functions in secondary prevention of disease in elderly clients
    a. Conduct a comprehensive health assessment of the elderly client, including an assessment of the client's body systems and status within the family and community
    b. Conduct community screening programs to detect health problems in elderly clients
    c. Educate the elderly client about treatments, therapies, and medication
    d. Supervise ancillary health care personnel who provide client services in the home
    e. Coordinate nursing services with those provided by other health team members
    f. Counsel the client and family as they adapt to life-style changes brought about by the client's health problems
    g. Help the client return to the best possible level of function
    h. Inform the client and family of appropriate community resources
    i. Promote a family and community network of support for the client
5. CHN functions in tertiary prevention of disease in elderly clients
    a. Initiate rehabilitation strategies during acute illness
    b. Assist the client with follow-up services in the home and community
    c. Coordinate nursing services with those provided by physical therapists, occupational therapists, speech therapists, and other health care providers
    d. Provide consultation services and education programs for individuals responsible for care of an elderly person

e. Support legislation and policies that address the concerns of elderly persons
f. Support a community network of support for elderly persons

O. Clients with chronic renal failure (CRF)

1. General information
   a. CRF is a progressive, irreversible deterioration of renal function; the body's ability to maintain metabolic and fluid and electrolyte balance fails, causing uremia and, ultimately, death
   b. CRF can develop insidiously over a number of years or can occur suddenly from acute renal failure
   c. CRF results in uremia and death unless treated by dialysis or by a kidney transplant
   d. Approximately 42,000 Americans die of irreversible kidney failure each year
2. CRF risk factors
   a. History of renal dysfunction
   b. History of uncontrolled hypertension
   c. History of diabetes
   d. Presence of hereditary disorders, such as polycystic kidney disease
   e. Vascular disorders
   f. Family history of renal disease
   g. Use of nephrotoxic drugs, such as aminoglycosides, gentamicin, tobramycin, colistimethate, polymyxin B, amphotericin B, vancomycin, amikacin, capreomycin, sulfonamides, phenacetin, radiologic contrast media, and thiazide diuretics
   h. Chronic analgesic abuse
   i. Exposure to toxic agents
   j. History of urinary tract infections
3. Population needs
   a. Available and accessible comprehensive home health services and community-based dialysis centers
   b. Well-coordinated home-based services for CRF clients and their families
   c. Direct treatment and management of the dysfunction
   d. Medication management
   e. Comprehensive, continuing client and family education about all aspects of dialysis treatment and kidney transplant follow-up care
   f. Client support services, including vocational rehabilitation and support groups
   g. Available and accessible kidneys for transplants
   h. Hospice services
4. CHN functions in primary prevention of CRF
   a. Teach individuals and community groups about kidney disease prevention, including preventing uncontrolled hypertension (using diet modification, exercise, medication, and other life-style management techniques), controlling diabetes (using diet modification, exercise, and

medication), avoiding or carefully controlling the use of potentially nephrotoxic drugs, and using proper hygiene to prevent urinary tract infections
   b. Monitor the home health care client who has an indwelling catheter, and minimize the risk of ascending infections and of further renal damage by removing the catheter as soon as possible
   c. Appraise the community's health status for specific renal problems and related needs
5. CHN functions in secondary prevention of CRF
   a. Screen individuals and community groups for diabetes and hypertension, with follow-up to ensure prompt diagnosis and treatment
   b. Teach the client about urinary tract infection symptoms and appropriate medical treatment
   c. Provide comprehensive home care for clients with CRF
   d. Teach the client and family about treatment aspects, including diet and fluid management, medications, infection prevention, and signs and symptoms of complications
   e. Counsel the client and family regarding short- and long-term disease management
   f. Support the client and family decision-making process regarding dialysis or a transplant
   g. Identify available community support groups for the client
6. CHN functions in tertiary prevention of CRF
   a. Provide comprehensive home care to clients receiving home- or institution-based dialysis
   b. Support the client and family as they adapt to life-style changes imposed by dialysis
   c. Help the client and family manage a home dialysis program
   d. Refer the client and family members to community services and organizations, such as the National Association of Patients on Hemodialysis and Transplantation
   e. Coordinate home health services with hospital or community dialysis center services
   f. Educate individuals and community groups regarding the crucial need for kidney donors
   g. Advocate accessible community services for CRF clients and their families
   h. Advocate a comprehensive, coordinated organ procurement program
   i. Counsel family members of prospective kidney donors regarding donation procedures and possible consequences

P. Clients with physical impairments
1. General information
   a. Approximately 35 million Americans are physically disabled to some degree; they constitute the largest U.S. minority group

b. About 12% of all children and youth are handicapped; 60% of these handicaps occurred after birth
c. Disability occurs in degrees—slight, moderate, severe, or total; primarily governed by the individual's ability to perform activities of daily living (ADLs) and be employed
d. Disability differs from handicap: disability is the degree of observable and measurable physical or mental impairment; handicap is the total readjustment necessitated by an impairment or disability that limits or prevents normal or useful functioning
e. Disability is classified as congenital or acquired, visible or invisible, stable or progressive
f. An individual can have a severe disability but be minimally handicapped—for example, a quadriplegic individual who maintains an active family role, runs a business, and drives a specially equipped van; an individual can be severely handicapped by a slight disability if unable to adjust to the disability and achieve a satisfying life-style
g. Some studies indicate that children with physical handicaps have a higher risk of abuse and neglect; other studies pinpoint abuse and neglect as causes of physical or mental handicaps
h. Adapting to the handicap—a complex process influenced by the individual, family, community, and social variables—is the most significant task facing a disabled individual and his family
i. Many handicaps are long term and require ongoing community resource utilization
j. Social attitudes have changed over the years, but handicapped individuals are still subjected to discrimination and prejudice

2. Possible physical impairment risk factors
   a. No known risk factors predispose an individual to physical impairment
   b. Conditions such as congenital malformations, child abuse and neglect, accidents, and systemic diseases have the potential to cause physical impairment
3. Population needs
   a. Assistance in redefining family roles, relationships, and division of labor
   b. Direct treatment and management of the disability or handicap
   c. Comprehensive community-based services to assist handicapped individuals and families with social, emotional, physical, and financial problems
   d. Access to comprehensive community resources and long-term care services
4. CHN functions in primary prevention of physical impairments
   a. Promote early and ongoing prenatal care to reduce the risk of congenital malformations

   b. Advocate community networks of prenatal services that target women with high-risk pregnancies, such as adolescents and those with low incomes
   c. Teach individuals and families about accident prevention in the home, school, and workplace
5. CHN functions in secondary prevention of physical impairments
   a. Provide direct comprehensive home care for clients recovering from disabling or handicapping conditions
   b. Support and counsel clients who have chronic illnesses to promote effective disease management and control
   c. Provide long-term support and counseling for the client and family to promote a positive family adaptation to the disability or handicap
   d. Support the family's efforts to promote the highest possible level of independence for the disabled or handicapped client
   e. Encourage the parents of a disabled child to avoid being overprotective, and promote growth and independence by teaching the child ADLs and other skills
   f. Help the client and family obtain community services that enhance adaptation
   g. Coordinate services provided in the client's home, including nursing care, physical therapy, occupational therapy, and speech therapy
   h. Help the family locate and obtain assistive devices for the disabled client
   i. Identify community agencies and resources useful to the client and family, such as support groups
   j. Inform the client and family about resource guides for handicapped or physically impaired individuals
   k. Help the family arrange respite services, when needed
6. CHN functions in tertiary prevention of physical impairments
   a. Coordinate services provided in the home or school with services provided by other community agencies
   b. Refer the client and family to appropriate community resources, such as vocational rehabilitation centers or family support groups that include siblings of handicapped children
   c. Advocate local, state, and federal policies that enrich the lives of disabled clients and their families
   d. Assist communities by consulting on or directly participating in the development of adequate resources for the physical, emotional, social, and financial needs of handicapped or disabled individuals, including transportation, vocational, and recreation services, community living arrangements, and respite care
   e. Promote programs that employ disabled individuals
   f. Demonstrate an acceptance of disabled individuals and their families

Q. Clients with seizure disorders

1. General information
   a. Approximately 4 million Americans have seizure disorders; incidence is highest in infants under age 1 and in individuals over age 55
   b. Seizure disorders may result from inborn errors of metabolism; any disease that affects the entire brain, such as electrolyte disturbances and infection or inflammation of the brain, its linings or blood vessels; poisons or drug reactions; degenerative nervous system disorders; tumors; allergic and immune reactions following viral infections; and immunizations.
   c. Approximately 60% of individuals with seizure disorders will become seizure-free with treatment; another 25% can achieve sufficient control to live functional, productive lives
   d. The remaining 15% cannot achieve consistent relief from symptoms; larger doses of anticonvulsant medication do not improve seizure control; daily life is adversely affected by seizure attacks and medication side effects
   e. Children with seizure disorders experience a higher rate of psychiatric disorders than unaffected children, probably caused by neurologic dysfunction
   f. Learning and school problems are more prevalent in children with seizure disorders
   g. Most children with seizure disorders have normal intelligence
2. Possible seizure disorder risk factors
   a. History of head injury
   b. Exposure to viral and bacterial infections
   c. Prolonged exposure to environmental pollutants, such as lead
   d. History of substance abuse
3. Population needs
   a. Lifelong access to comprehensive community health care services
   b. Support networks in the home, school, and workplace
   c. Acceptance by the general public as normal, functioning individuals
   d. Medication management
   e. Health education
   f. Direct treatment of the dysfunction
4. CHN functions in primary prevention of seizure disorders
   a. Identify clients at risk in the community (case-finding)
   b. Refer pregnant women at risk for early and continuing prenatal care, with follow-up care for the infant
   c. Advocate accessible well-child services provided by doctors, nurses, and other practitioners associated with private, voluntary, and official agencies
   d. Teach clients and community groups about accident prevention, emphasizing head protection during activities that present a risk of head injury, such as skateboarding and bicycling

   e. Provide parents with health guidance about treating symptoms of fever and infections in children at home, including guidelines for seeking medical attention
   f. Support community initiatives to reduce sources of lead, such as removing lead-based paint from older housing
5. CHN functions in secondary prevention of seizure disorders
   a. Counsel the client and family to resolve any feelings of shame, guilt, or embarrassment
   b. Educate parents about the problem's nature and scope, about medication management (including therapeutic and adverse side effects), and about the need to treat the child as normal
   c. Help the family understand seizure disorder etiology and treatment and develop a positive attitude toward the affected child
   d. Encourage positive parenting behaviors
   e. Educate teachers and other school personnel about the care of school-age children with seizure disorders, including measures for handling a seizure at school
   f. Provide ongoing physical, social, and developmental assessment of the client and provide the appropriate family guidance
   g. Support family efforts to help the client develop normally
   h. Teach family members how to respond to seizures at home
6. CHN functions in tertiary prevention of seizure disorders
   a. Promote supportive home and school climates to help the child or adolescent with a seizure disorder master developmental tasks
   b. Refer the parents of a child experiencing social or learning problems to appropriate community resources
   c. Refer the client and family to appropriate community agencies, including support groups
   d. Advocate community education and vocation opportunities for clients with seizure disorders

R. Clients with multiple sclerosis (MS)

1. General information
   a. MS is a chronic, frequently progressive, disease of the central nervous system characterized by small patches of demyelination in the spinal cord and brain that results in nerve transmission disorder
   b. The cause of MS is unknown; however, myelin damage that results from a viral infection early in life probably compromises immune responses later in life
   c. MS is more common in people living in northern climates
   d. Women develop MS twice as often as men
   e. Individuals with MS experience unpredictable exacerbations and remissions

f. The degree of MS disability varies; some never experience disability, others experience mild and temporary disability; in some, the disease is arrested; and only a small number become severely disabled and bedridden
g. MS is considered the most disabling neurologic disease of adults in the 20 to 40 age-group; is called "the great crippler of young adults"; and, after arthritis and trauma, is the chief cause of disability in adults of working age
h. MS symptom areas and associated incidence rates are motor and movement, 35%; touch, 35%; vision, 20%; other (bladder, bowel, brain), 10%
i. Individuals with MS may have temporary episodes of immobility following an exacerbation, but aggressive management frequently restores mobility; about 75% experience prolonged remissions and remain ambulatory
j. Early onset of MS increases individual and family medical, psychological, social, and economic problems

2. Possible MS risk factors
   a. Family history of MS
   b. Environment: living in urban areas or cold, damp climates
   c. Sex: occurs more frequently in women
   d. Economic status: occurs more frequently in higher socioeconomic classes
3. Population needs
   a. Comprehensive community services, such as home health services, physical therapy, and counseling and other mental health services to help victims and their families manage exacerbations
   b. Available comprehensive rehabilitation services, including physical and vocational resources
   c. Health education
   d. Illness management during exacerbations
4. CHN functions in primary prevention of MS
   a. Provide community education programs about the illness to individuals, families, and community groups
   b. Appraise the community's health status by examining MS epidemiologic data
5. CHN functions in secondary prevention of MS
   a. Provide direct care in the client's home during exacerbations, including promoting rest and stress avoidance, keeping the client cool with baths or ice packs, giving regular passive range-of-motion exercises when the client is confined to bed, and teaching the client and family how to administer steroids or other prescribed medications
   b. Supervise home health aides and other ancillary personnel providing home health care
   c. Help the client and family cope with the stress imposed by increased disability

   d. Teach the client and family general MS management measures to prevent exacerbations, such as eating a balanced diet, maintaining desirable body weight, avoiding infections (especially urinary tract infections), and exercising moderately to maintain the highest activity level possible
   e. Teach relaxation and coordination exercises in the home to promote physical mobility
   f. Assess the home for safety features and hazards and make appropriate recommendations to the family
   g. Help the client choose and acquire appropriate assistive devices and instruct the client in their use
   h. Teach the client and family how to avoid client injury when motor dysfunction causes incoordination and clumsiness
6. CHN functions in tertiary prevention of MS
   a. Coordinate nursing services with other health professionals, such as physical therapists, occupational therapists, and speech therapists, to enhance client rehabilitation
   b. Promote rehabilitation of the client's bladder and bowel control by teaching the family to manage fluids, provide a high-fiber diet, and institute a bowel training program, if necessary
   c. Counsel the client and family about adapting to the disease and its limitations, including emotional changes, such as depression and denial
   d. Counsel the client and family regarding all aspects of adapting to the illness, including alternatives for providing care and maintaining a positive, hopeful attitude
   e. Counsel the client and partner about problems that may interfere with sexual activity; refer the couple to a sex counselor, if necessary
   f. Refer the client to appropriate community resources, including support groups and vocational rehabilitation services

S. Clients with dementia

1. General information
   a. Dementia refers to a group of symptoms characterized by memory loss and an inability to think and reason clearly; some dementias are reversible, such as those caused by thyroid disease; others are irreversible and progressive, such as Alzheimer's disease and multi-infarct dementia
   b. Alzheimer's disease is characterized by structural changes in the brain, including brain atrophy; it appears to be the most frequent cause of irreversible dementia in adults
   c. Multi-infarct dementia is a series of strokes within the brain; the second most common cause of irreversible dementia
   d. Elderly individuals who experience gradual memory impairment and intellectual decline may have Alzheimer's disease
   e. Between 5% and 6% of Americans age 65 and older, or 1.5 million individuals, have Alzheimer's disease

f. Incidence increases with age; 15% to 20% of the elderly population is affected by age 85
g. Approximately half of all U.S. admissions to long-term care facilities are caused by Alzheimer's disease
h. Life expectancy decreases for individuals with Alzheimer's disease, depending on the age of onset
i. The course of Alzheimer's disease is 2 to 20 years, with the terminal stage about 5 years after initial symptoms
j. Little is understood about the disease, and no specific treatment exists
k. The effects of the disease on the family and caregivers is profound as the individual gradually loses physical, psychological, and social function

2. Possible dementia risk factors
   a. Since the cause of dementia is unknown, no risk factors can be identified
   b. Alzheimer's disease is associated with advancing age but is not a consequence of the aging process
3. Population needs
   a. Extensive research into the cause and treatment of Alzheimer's disease and related dementias
   b. Supportive community services, such as adult day-care and home health care
   c. Support services in the community for family members and other caregivers
   d. Available and accessible long-term care facilities
4. CHN functions in primary prevention of dementia
   a. Provide education programs in the community on the problems of dementias
   b. Participate in research and epidemiologic data gathering to identify causes and risk factors
5. CHN functions in secondary prevention of dementia
   a. Provide support for family members and caregivers as they cope with the physical and mental changes in the client while treating the client with dignity
   b. Teach the family and caregivers how to assist the client who has limited ability to participate in self-care, including assisting with dressing and hygiene, allowing the client to sleep at will and expecting irregular sleep patterns, expecting the confused client to use any available container or the floor for elimination, avoiding medications in large capsules or tablets, and expecting client withdrawal and isolation
   c. Help the family and caregivers understand the disease consequences as deterioration progresses
   d. Inform the family about educational resources and support groups, such as the Alzheimer's Disease and Related Disorders Association and the Alzheimer's Support Group; books about Alzheimer's disease written for general audiences often help family members understand and cope with a family member with Alzheimer's disease

6. CHN functions in tertiary prevention of dementia
   a. Refer family members to supportive community groups, such as adult day-care centers, family support groups, and respite services
   b. When necessary, counsel and support the family in their decision to place the client in a long-term care facility
   c. Advocate a substantial expansion of long-term care resources
   d. Advocate comprehensive, interdisciplinary services for persons with Alzheimer's disease and their families

T. Clients with CVA

1. General information
   a. CVA, or stroke, is the third most common cause of death in the United States following heart disease and cancer
   b. Approximately 85,000 individuals die each year from CVAs; another 1 million survive but are disabled
   c. Thrombosis, a clot lodged in an artery or vein, is the most common cause of stroke and is usually caused by atherosclerosis
   d. Incidence of CVA has declined during the past 30 years; however, CVA continues to be the most frequent neurologic cause of hospital admission and a major cause of referral for home health care
2. Possible CVA risk factors
   a. Age: risk increases with age
   b. Family history of cerebrovascular disease
   c. History of cardiac or vascular disease: a history of hypertension, hypercholesterolemia, cardiac disease, or atherosclerosis increases risk
   d. History of diabetes
   e. Smoking
   f. Oral contraceptive use
3. Population needs
   a. Available and accessible health care resources for prompt CVA treatment
   b. Comprehensive community-based rehabilitation services
   c. Community education programs to promote behaviors that decrease the risk of CVA
   d. Direct treatment and management of the illness
4. CHN functions in primary prevention of CVA
   a. Educate individuals of all ages about heart disease and hypertension prevention; measures include a diet low in sodium and cholesterol, proper body weight, not smoking, and regular exercise
   b. Help clients with diabetes mellitus control the disease using medication, diet, and exercise
   c. Teach hypertensive clients how to control the disease using diet, medication, exercise, stress reduction, and giving up smoking
   d. Teach female clients of childbearing age about alternatives to oral contraceptives, especially women age 35 and older, those with hypertension, or those who smoke

5. CHN functions in secondary prevention of CVA
   a. Provide direct care in the client's home following discharge from the hospital
   b. Teach family members all aspects of the physical and emotional care of CVA victims, including dealing with motor function loss, speech loss, perceptual disturbances, mental activity impairment and psychological effects, and bladder dysfunction
   c. Support the client and family as they adapt to the client's disability state; encourage them to work with the client's strengths and potential
   d. Supervise ancillary personnel providing care in the home, such as home health aides
   e. Help the client and family institute a rehabilitation program
   f. Help the family choose, purchase, and learn to operate any necessary assistive devices for the client
   g. Identify appropriate community resources for the client and family
6. CHN functions in tertiary prevention of CVA
   a. Coordinate the activities of the interdisciplinary home health team involved in the client's rehabilitation, including physical therapists, speech therapists, occupational therapists, and social workers
   b. Support the client and family throughout rehabilitation
   c. Refer the client and family to appropriate community resources, including vocational rehabilitation

Points to Remember

The community health nurse should know the risk factors associated with each high-risk population and know which factors can be modified.

The community health nurse should be aware of interventions useful in reducing, modifying, or eliminating selected risk factors.

Nursing responsibilities for high-risk populations include efforts in primary, secondary, and tertiary levels of prevention.

Promoting the health of individuals in high-risk populations and their families improves the health of the community as a whole.

Glossary

Demyelination—destruction of myelin, the fatty and protein material that sheathes certain nerve fibers in the brain and spinal cord

Dialysis—differential diffusion of solute through a semipermeable membrane separating two solutions

Extended care facility—a type of long-term care facility for short-term, posthospital discharge clients

Long-term care—client attention usually provided in institutional settings that range from custodial care to skilled nursing care 24 hours each day; in general, a skilled nursing care facility offers care under the supervision of a licensed nurse 24 hours a day; an intermediate care facility provides less nursing care

Risk factors—characteristic or exposure that precedes disease development and has a high correlation with increased rates of disease, antisocial behavior, or disability; may be causative factors

Uremia—excess urea and other nitrogenous wastes in the blood

SECTION XI

The U.S. Health Care Delivery System and Community Health

Learning Objectives

After studying this section, the reader should be able to:

- Describe the historical development of the U.S. health care delivery system.
- Trace the development of official and voluntary agencies.
- Describe the basic organizational structure of the health care delivery system.
- Discuss facets of selected legislation related to community health care.
- Describe the financing mechanisms for community health care.
- Discuss the impact of health care financing on community health.

XI. The U.S. Health Care Delivery System and Community Health

A. Developmental perspectives

1. 1800 to 1899
   a. Infectious disease epidemics affected large population segments
   b. Health problems stemmed from contaminated food and water, inadequate sewage disposal, and poor housing conditions
   c. Most individuals under hospital care died; most individuals were cared for at home by family and friends
2. 1900 to 1945
   a. Acute infectious diseases affecting large population segments were brought under control; epidemics were significantly reduced
   b. Environmental conditions improved markedly with major advances in water purification, sanitary sewage disposal, milk quality, and urban housing quality
   c. Health care problems shifted from epidemics to individual acute infections or traumatic episodes
3. 1946 to present day
   a. Acute infectious health problems are well controlled
   b. Health care focus shifted to chronic health problems, such as heart disease, cancer, diabetes, stroke, and circulatory disorders

B. Historical perspectives

1. Official (government) agency development
   a. Early community health care consisted of private practice with little government involvement
   b. First formal federal government intervention was the Marine Hospital Service Act of 1798, which subsidized medical and hospital care for disabled seamen
   c. Official community health care agencies first emerged at the local government level during the late 1700s and early 1800s
   d. "Report of the Sanitary Commission of Massachusetts," written by Lemuel Shattuck in 1850 and known as the Shattuck Report, described public health concepts and methods; used as a foundation for today's public health service; advocated state and local health boards, environmental sanitation, collection and use of vital statistics, systematic disease studies, food and drug production controls, urban planning, training schools for nurses, and preventive medicine
   e. First state board of health, later called the department of health, was formed in Massachusetts in 1869
   f. First full-time county health departments were established in North Carolina and Washington in 1911
   g. Marine Service Hospital became the U.S. Public Health Service in 1912
   h. National Institutes of Health (NIH) were founded in 1912
   i. Communicable Disease Center, later known as the National Centers for Disease Control (CDC), was established in 1940

j. National Office of Vital Statistics, later known as the National Center for Health Statistics, was formed in 1940
k. Federal agencies became organized under the Department of Health, Education, and Welfare in 1953; later reorganized as the Department of Health and Human Services (DHHS)

ORGANIZATIONAL CHART OF THE DEPARTMENT OF HEALTH AND HUMAN SERVICES

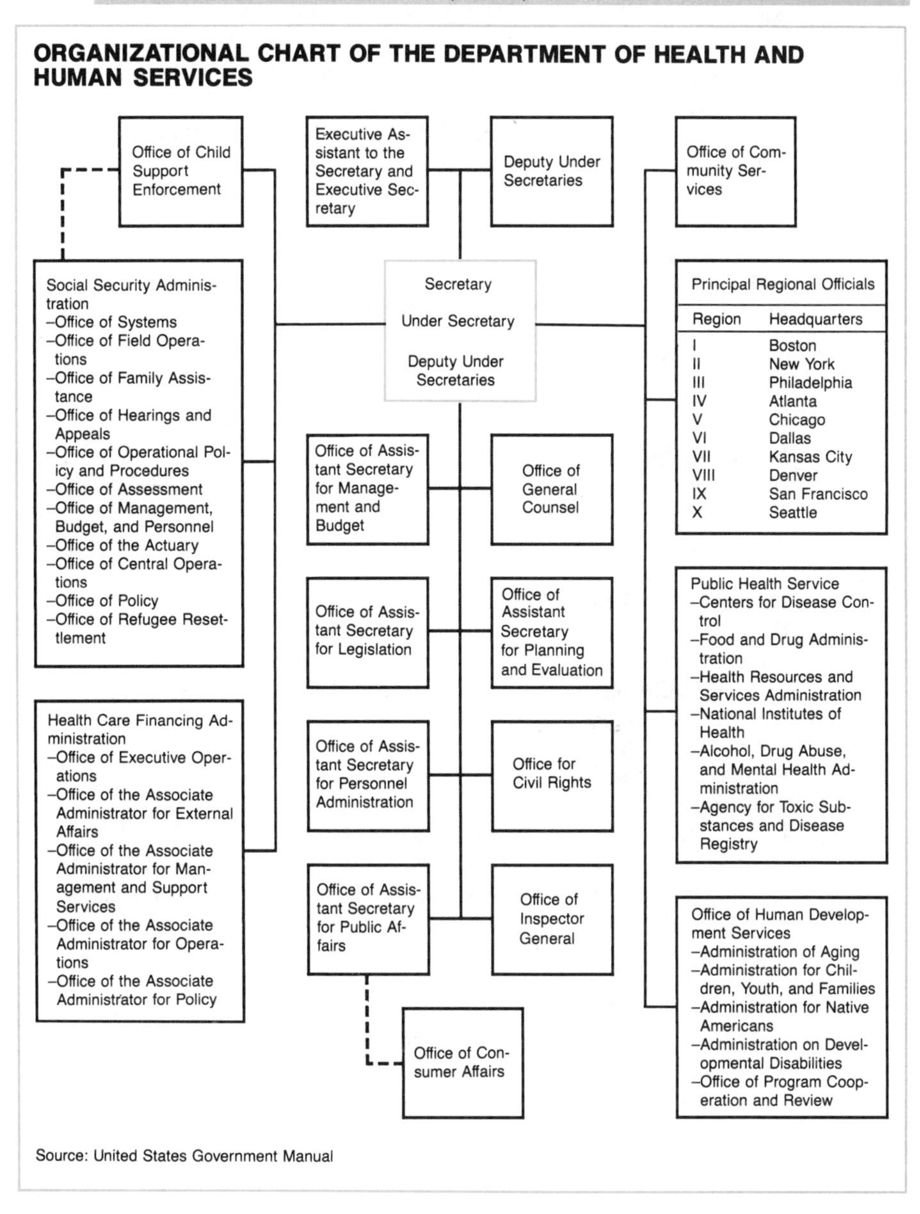

Source: United States Government Manual

2. Voluntary (private) agency development
   a. First voluntary agencies were formed in the late 1800s
   b. American Public Health Association was founded in 1872
   c. Anti-Tuberculosis Society of Philadelphia, founded in 1892, was the first voluntary health agency
   d. American Red Cross was officially established in 1889
   e. National Society for the Prevention of Blindness was created in 1908
   f. Mental Health Association was established in 1909
   g. American Cancer Society was founded in 1913
   h. National Easter Seal Society for Crippled Children and Adults was founded in 1921
   i. Planned Parenthood Federation was formed in 1921

C. Types of health care agencies

1. Official agencies
   a. Established by law; are *government* agencies
   b. Coordinate activities best carried out by communitywide action
   c. Provide health-related and welfare services, including public works, police and fire services, agricultural services, and housing authority services
   d. Funded by federal tax dollars
   e. Can be affiliated with local, state, or federal governments; for example, city, county, and state health departments; state hospitals; Environmental Protection Agency (EPA); U.S. Public Health Service; NIH
2. Voluntary agencies
   a. Governed by a board of directors; are *nonprofit* agencies
   b. Formed by individuals or groups to address a specific health service need; often focused on one population group or disease
   c. Provide health services to a large number of individuals in various settings; may augment official agency services
   d. Include research and education activities
   e. Funded by contributions, gifts, endowments, and some third-party payments
   f. Exempt from federal and state income taxes
   g. Exist at the *local level*—for example, the visiting nurse association and city or county mental health associations; *state level*—for example, the state cancer society and state heart association; or *national level*—for example, the American Diabetes Association and American Red Cross
3. Proprietary agencies
   a. Operated *for profit;* governed by the agency owner
   b. Provide direct health care services, promote health care delivery by establishing and enforcing professional practice standards, provide education, and conduct research

c. Funded by third-party payments, owner's capital, and membership fees
d. Not exempt from federal taxes
e. Include private, independent providers, such as medical group practices, some hospitals and institutions, and home care agencies

D. Organization of health care services

1. Local health agencies
   a. Basic unit for delivering public health services to a specific geographic area
   b. Functions include assessing the public's health status and needs, determining whether needs are met, and coordinating information from the state and federal levels
   c. Services include community health, environmental health, mental health, and personal health
2. State health agencies
   a. Provide public health leadership and monitor state health needs and services
   b. Functions include statewide health planning, coordinating intergovernmental and interstate agency relations, and setting and regulating statewide health policies and standards
   c. Services include personal health, environmental health, laboratory services, occupational health, communicable disease control, maintenance of vital statistics, health education, training, and research
3. Federal health agencies
   a. These provide for the population's general welfare as stipulated in the Preamble to the U.S. Constitution
   b. Functions include personal health and welfare, international health and welfare, planning of health and welfare services, policy making, health education, training, and research
   c. The DHHS, the primary federal health agency, contains the Social Security Agency, Office of Child Support Enforcement, Office of Community Services, Office of Human Development Services, Health Care Financing Administration, and Public Health Service
   d. The Public Health Service contains the CDC, Food and Drug Administration (FDA), Health Resources and Services Administration, NIH, Agency for Toxic Substances and Disease Registry, and Alcohol, Drug Abuse, and Mental Health Administration
   e. Other federal health agencies include the Department of Agriculture, the Department of Commerce, and the EPA

E. Legislation significant to community health services

1. Children's Health Bureau Act of 1912
   a. Provided federal support for efforts to reduce the mortality rates of mothers and infants
   b. Reduced infant mortality rate between 1915 and 1928 by 33%

2. Sheppard-Towner Act of 1921
   a. Expanded the Children's Health Bureau functions; provided for communication of health information between the federal and state government and among the states as well
   b. Provided federal funding for the state administration of programs to promote infant health and welfare
   c. Established a model for later health and welfare programs for maternal and child health
3. Social Security Act of 1935
   a. Established welfare insurance and assistance programs
   b. Established benefits for poor and elderly people, and crippled children
   c. Started financial assistance to state and local agencies providing public health services
4. Food, Drug, and Cosmetic Act of 1938
   a. Created the FDA
   b. Established in response to mounting concern over food and drug additives and unsanitary food processing practices
5. Hill-Burton Act of 1946
   a. Linked public health planning to specific needs in the population—a first legislative effort
   b. Provided states with hospital construction funds
   c. Tied funding to the formation of state planning councils that document the need for new facilities
   d. Required that hospitals built under this act dedicate a portion of their beds to indigent clients
6. Heart Disease, Cancer, and Stroke Amendments of 1965
   a. Established regional medical programs
   b. Was one of the first legislative efforts in comprehensive health planning
   c. Encouraged local participation in health planning
   d. Funded program planning and operation
7. Social Security Act Amendments of 1965
   a. Established Medicare as a federal health insurance program for individuals over age 65 and on social security, the disabled, and individuals with end-stage renal disease requiring dialysis
   b. Covered hospitalization (Part A) and doctor care and other health-related services (Part B, supplementary)
   c. Established Medicaid as a joint federal and state assistance program for low-income individuals and their families and medically indigent individuals (those with high medical expenses); attempted to provide the poor with better medical care by paying for this care
8. Comprehensive Health Planning and Public Health Service Amendments Act of 1966
   a. Promoted further advances in comprehensive health planning
   b. Established comprehensive health planning agencies
   c. Integrated many categorical health and research efforts into one system

   d. Emphasized comprehensive health planning at local, state, and regional levels
   e. Sought to improve the efficiency and effectiveness of health care while containing costs
9. Health Manpower Act of 1968
   a. Increased the number of health care personnel by providing educational institutions with funds for construction, training, special projects, student loans, and scholarships
   b. Replaced several acts that had similar goals but fragmented approaches
10. Occupational Safety and Health Act of 1970
   a. Provided worker protection against personal injury or illness resulting from hazardous working conditions
   b. Dealt with workers' compensation, toxic substance control, and access to employee exposure and medical records
11. Professional Standards and Review Organization (PSRO) Amendment to the Social Security Act (1972)
   a. Sought cost containment and improved quality of care
   b. Created autonomous organizations, not affiliated with hospitals or ambulatory care agencies, to monitor and review the quality of care provided to Medicare and Medicaid patients
   c. Created PSRO review boards, composed primarily of doctors, to examine the need for care, length of stay, and quality of care and then compare findings with locally developed standards; PSROs had to address the major problem of a lack of universally accepted criteria and standards common to all areas
12. Health Maintenance Organization (HMO) Act of 1973
   a. Added federal support to the idea of prospective payment for medical care
   b. Authorized funding for feasibility studies, planning, grants, and loans to stimulate growth in qualifying HMOs
   c. Sought to introduce competition into the area of health care payment
   d. Required a business employing 25 or more individuals to offer an HMO health insurance option when such options were available locally
13. National Health Planning and Resource Development Act of 1974
   a. Consolidated federal, state, and regional health planning efforts under one program to improve comprehensive health planning regulation and evaluation by facilitating intergovernmental cooperation
   b. Stressed the need for consumer involvement in health planning
   c. Established agencies within the health care delivery system and at the state level to help identify national health priorities and facilitate state and regional health planning
14. Health Professionals Education Assistance Act of 1976
   a. Sought to balance the supply of health professionals with the country's need for health care
   b. Created education incentives to draw more doctors into rural practices

15. Social Security Amendments of 1983
    a. Addressed spiraling health care costs
    b. Sought to promote a focus on client care that emphasized results and to contain health costs while maintaining the quality of care
    c. Shifted health care payment from *retrospective* to *prospective*
    d. Established a schedule for Medicare hospital payments according to a preestablished fixed rate based on discharge diagnosis; known as Diagnosis-Related Groups
    e. Permitted hospitals with costs less than the Medicare reimbursement to keep the difference; hospitals with costs that exceeded the amount reimbursed had to absorb the difference
    f. Provided an incentive to reduce health care costs
16. Catastrophic Health Care Act of 1988
    a. Established unlimited health care expense coverage after the client met a specific annual deductible amount
    b. Placed a ceiling on out-of-pocket expenses for services covered under Medicare (Part B)
    c. Established cost sharing of outpatient drug expenses after the client met a specific annual deductible amount
    d. Expanded skilled nursing facility and home health care benefits
    e. Removed the limit on number of days for respite hospice care

F. Health care financing for community health

1. Third-party payment
    a. Health care provider receives reimbursement from an individual or organization other than the client for services rendered to that client

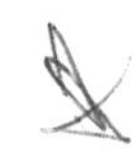

    b. Payers include private insurance companies such as Blue Cross and Blue Shield, Aetna, and Prudential; independent health plans such as HMOs and self-insurance plans; and government health programs such as Medicare and Medicaid
2. Direct payment
    a. Client pays for health care necessities
    b. Payment covers health care expenses by the client with no health insurance; payment for partial services, such as doctor's office visits and prescriptions; and payment of deductible amount before third-party reimbursement
3. Voluntary support
    a. Direct or indirect funding benefits clients who may otherwise go without health services
    b. Support includes donation of funds for programs and donation of an individual's time and service
4. CHN implications
    a. Demonstrate an awareness of the health care financing options available in the community

b. Use a knowledge of financing options when working with individuals, families, and community groups
c. Provide cost-effective, quality nursing care in the community setting
d. Help the client understand community health financing programs

G. Issues and trends in health care service delivery

1. Impact of financing on community health practice
   a. Incentives for illness care services created disincentives for the efficient use of resources
   b. Retrospective reimbursement encouraged spending
   c. Tax-deductible employer contributions for health care coverage encouraged spending
   d. Nontaxable employee health benefits encouraged spending
   e. Spending limitations for illness care caused an overall reduction in funds available for public health
   f. Increased private sector competition caused the reorganization of traditional community health agencies
2. Trends in health care financing
   a. An expanding federal role in health care service financing and regulation
   b. Escalating health care costs
   c. Stronger cost containment efforts
   d. An expanding role for HMOs as a cost containment approach
   e. Continuing efforts to develop national health insurance
   f. Continuing use of *prospective* payment plans
   g. Increasing competition in the health care industry; some health care delivery organizations will not survive the increasing competition and financial pressure
3. Trends in the delivery of health care services
   a. Selective hospitalization, with an increasing emphasis on ambulatory care services
   b. Shorter hospital stays with sicker patients being discharged for care at home
   c. Increasing deinstitutionalization of clients with chronic conditions, such as mental illness, mental retardation, and immobilizing physical problems
   d. Increasing numbers of elderly clients requiring services for chronic, rather than acute, health problems
   e. Increasing emphasis on illness prevention and health promotion services and on nutrition and fitness
   f. Expanding consumer knowledge and sophistication because of increased health care provider options
   g. Changes in the structure and pattern of services as technologic advances help save lives that previously could not be saved
   h. Development of alternative health care delivery methods to reduce costs and promote competition
   i. Expansion in services provided by the community
   j. Emergence of self-care and risk reduction as central philosophic concepts in health care delivery

4. Ethical issues for community health professionals caused by trends in health care financing and service delivery
   a. Allocating scarce financial and human resources; deciding which client groups will receive service when not all can be served
   b. Addressing ethical dilemmas posed by advanced technologic capabilities, such as determining who should receive the benefit of the technology and at what cost
5. CHN implications
   a. Pursue nursing research to generate knowledge that guides practice in promoting client health and well-being; prevent health problems that can reduce client productivity and satisfaction; decrease the impact of an illness on the client's coping skills, productivity, and general satisfaction; ensure that the health care needs of vulnerable groups are met with appropriate strategies; design and develop health care systems that meet the community's needs in a cost-effective manner; promote health, well-being, and personal health competency for clients of all ages; and validate the effectiveness of nursing interventions
   b. Consider cost-effective and efficient methods of delivering services, such as group interventions
   c. Consider using the media for health information delivery
   d. Assume a leadership role in illness prevention and health promotion
   e. Develop means for making CHN an integral component of the health care agency and health care system
   f. Develop and maintain more control in the management and delivery of CHN services
   g. Participate in studies and other efforts to determine the costs and scope of nursing services
   h. Participate actively in policy making and engage in political action to get policies implemented
   i. Participate in political decision making at federal, state, and local levels to influence health care policy and service development
   j. Develop marketing skills and strategies to provide cost-effective, responsive care by involving clients in the care process, providing additional services based on those the target group desires, increasing the nurse's accessibility to clients, conducting systematic outreach and follow-up, providing convenient service hours and waiting times, employing members from target groups, and reducing restrictive eligibility requirements
   k. Participate in the political process by learning about the political and legislative process, communicating with legislators and monitoring their performance on health issues, informing legislators about relevant health issues, joining political action committees, advocating desirable changes in laws and policies affecting nursing practice and community health, assuming community leadership positions, and becoming involved in community coalition groups with similar community health interests

Points to Remember

The network of community health services has evolved over a long period of this country's history.

Community health services are provided by official, voluntary, and proprietary agencies.

The federal role in health care planning has been severely reduced over the years.

Cost containment has become a crucial consideration in health care service delivery.

Community health nurses can participate in the promotion of sound community health policies and health services in many ways.

Glossary

Deductible—the dollar amount of health care service expense paid by an insured individual before his insurance coverage takes over payment responsibility

Health maintenance organizations (HMOs)—groups that provide prepaid, comprehensive health care services to participants for a monthly premium

Medically indigent—individuals unable to afford a catastrophic illness or acute crisis but who are above the poverty level and can afford basic necessities

Prospective payment—system in which health care payment rates are established prior to care delivery rather than after care delivery

Third-party payment—a health services reimbursement source that is not directly associated with the client or service provider

Appendix

Selected community health organization resources

Administration on Aging
Department of Health and Human Services
330 Independence Avenue, S.W.
Washington, D.C. 20201

American Association for Maternal
and Child Health, Inc.
P.O. Box 965
Los Altos, Calif. 94022

American Association for Vital Records
and Public Health Statistics
c/o Utah Department of Health
P.O. Box 2500
Salt Lake City, Utah 84110

American Cancer Society, Inc.
777 Third Avenue
New York, N.Y. 10017

American Diabetes Association
600 Fifth Avenue
New York, N.Y. 10020

American Epilepsy Society
38238 Glenn Avenue
Willoughby, Ohio 44094

American Foundation for the Blind
15 West 16th Street
New York, N.Y. 10011

American Heart Association
7320 Greenville Avenue
Dallas, Tex. 75231

American Lung Association
1740 Broadway
New York, N.Y. 10019

American Mental Health Foundation, Inc.
2 East 86th Street
New York, NY 10028

American Nurses' Association
Council on Gerontological Nursing
2420 Pershing Road
Kansas City, Mo. 64108

American Red Cross
17th and D Streets, N.W.
Washington, D.C. 20006

Arthritis Foundation
3400 Peachtree Road, N.E.
Atlanta, Ga. 30326

Goodwill Industries of America, Inc.
9200 Wisconsin Avenue
Washington, D.C. 20014

Gray Panthers
3635 Chestnut Street
Philadelphia, Pa. 19104

Health and Education Resources
4733 Bethesda Avenue, Suite 735
Bethesda, Md. 20014

International Childbirth Education
Association, Inc.
8635 Fremont Avenue South
Minneapolis, Minn. 55420

International Council on Health,
Physical Education, and Recreation
1201 16th Street, N.W., Room 417
Washington, D.C. 20036

The Juvenile Diabetes Foundation
23 East 26th Street
New York, N.Y. 10010

La Leche League International, Inc.
9616 Minneapolis Avenue
Franklin Park, Ill. 60131

Leukemia Society of America, Inc.
800 Second Avenue
New York, N.Y. 10017

March of Dimes Birth Defects Foundation
1275 Mamaroneck Avenue
White Plains, N.Y. 10605

Mental Health Association
National Headquarters
1800 North Kent Street
Arlington, Va. 22209

Muscular Dystrophy Association
810 Seventh Avenue, 27th Floor
New York, N.Y. 10019

National Committee for the Prevention
of Alcoholism and Drug Dependency
6830 Laurel Street, N.W.
Washington, D.C. 20012

National Council on Alcoholism, Inc.
733 Third Avenue
New York, N.Y. 10017

National Council on Drug Abuse
571 West Jackson Boulevard
Chicago, Ill. 60606

National Council on Health Care Services
1200 15th Street, N.W., Suite 601
Washington, D.C. 20005

The National Hemophilia Foundation
25 West 39th Street
New York, N.Y. 10018

National Institute on Aging
Building 31C, 9000 Rockville Pike
Bethesda, Md. 20205

OSHA
200 Constitution Avenue, N.W.
Washington, D.C. 20210

Planned Parenthood Federation
of America, Inc.
810 Seventh Avenue
New York, N.Y. 10019

United Cerebral Palsy Association, Inc.
66 East 34th Street
New York, N.Y. 10016

Index

t refers to a table.

F

G

H

IJK

L

M

N

O

P

QR

S

T

UV

WXYZ

t refers to a table.

Notes

Notes

Notes

Notes

Notes

Notes